Stoma Care

Evidence-based Guideline on Stoma Care in the Netherlands

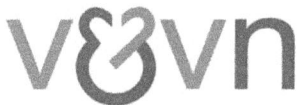

v&vn

Beroepsvereniging van zorgprofessionals

Stomaverpleegkundigen

V&VN Department of Stoma Care Nurses
6 November 2012

Evidence-based Guideline on Stoma Care in the Netherlands

Authors:
Mrs. J.J.G. Smelt MANP

Mrs. H.G. Baas
Mr. H. Beekhuizen
Mrs. T. Bremer-Goossens
Mrs. J.E.C. de Buck VS
Mrs. M. Broekhof
Mrs. M.P. den Hertog
Mrs. M.A. Klievink VS
Mrs. S.I. Klok
Mrs. I.M. Mast
Mrs. J.H. Rook

6 November 2012

ISBN/EAN: 978-90-820895-0-9

The Dutch guideline can be accessed on the website: http://stomaverpleegkunde.venvn.nl
Please contact V&VN Department of Stoma Care Nurses for any questions regarding the contents of this guideline.

Foreword

I proudly present this Dutch Guideline on Stoma Care on behalf of V&VN Department of Stoma Care Nurses. I am very pleased with this guideline and I hope that this document will bring more uniformity in the provision of stoma care in hospitals. That this is currently not the case has been shown by the research done by the Dutch Ostomy Association, and is also evident in the in the Stoma Care Guideline.

Another reason why I am pleased with this guideline is that it provides stoma patients with clear information about stoma care. For patients to feel in control of their situation, it is crucial that they have access to correct information.

This edition is especially intended for stoma care nurses. The guideline shows that stoma care is a specialised expertise and requires specific knowledge and experience. In my view this guideline is an outstanding account of the knowledge on stoma care to date. You, the stoma care nurse, can be proud of this!

What is the purpose of this document? The Dutch Ostomy Association hopes that you will actively use this guideline in your work. Whilst improving your work, you will be creating greater uniformity in stoma care. Personally I hope that this guideline will also be applied when making financial decisions on stoma care.

This guideline will help to improve stoma care and therefore also the quality of life of stoma patients. And that is exactly what you and the Dutch Ostomy Association aspire to achieve! I wish you all the best with the implementation of this stoma care guideline.

Thijs Fonville
Chairman Nederlandse Stomavereniging (Dutch Ostomy Association)

Table of contents

Introduction

Purpose and target group

This document is the first Dutch evidence-based guideline on stoma care. The purpose of this guideline is to increase the quality of stoma care in the Netherlands through uniformity.
This guideline is directed at nurses and care providers. It can also be used by patients, the Dutch Ostomy Association as well as other occupational groups.
The working group chose to focus on the incontinent stomata (colostomy, ileostomy and urostomy) in adults over the age of 18. Continent stomata as well as children with a stoma are not addressed in this guideline because of the specific nature of stoma care for these groups. Neither will general pre- and postoperative care aspects such as laxative, shaving and nutritional policies, be discussed. Only where these aspects are directly related to stoma care, they will be mentioned. It is needless to say that this guideline is about nursing care. Medical aspects are beyond the scope of this guideline.

Background and motivation

The development of this guideline is carried out on behalf of the board of V&VN Department of Stoma Care Nurses. The V&VN is the umbrella organization for nurses and care providers in the Netherlands. The professional association for stoma care nurses (formerly VVSN, now V&VN Department of Stoma Care Nurses) was established in 1985. Since then, many nurses have worked towards increasing the quality of stoma care by describing operations and techniques in manuals and protocols.
It is commonly known that these manuals should ideally be supported and substantiated by medical and scientific literature, which in turn is based on excellent medical evidence. Although the specialists' or expert's opinion is still considered valuable, it is no longer considered to be solely sufficient as a basis for professional care. This is, amongst others, one of the reasons why the V&VN has expressed the ambition to compile an evidence-based guideline. Within the association, several committees are working on sub-assignments and the "committee technique" has been put in charge of developing the evidence-based guideline.
In 2009 the members of the technique committee (hereafter referred to as the working group) followed a two day training course on how to develop an evidence-based guideline. This was regarded as the starting point for this document and scientific support was available at all times to the members of the committee.

The main objective of the V&VN is the "development and promotion of stoma care in the broadest sense" (www.vvsn.com/page/Welkom).
The V&VN Department aims to achieve this by "developing protocols, initiating scientific research, developing a uniform conceptual framework and co-operating in various trainings which are linked to all possible levels on which stoma care nurses practice". For this an evidence-based guideline is necessary.

The working group members want to emphasise that compiling this guideline would have been impossible without the co-operation of several other parties. For this the working group wants to express her gratitude. Mrs. G. Bours primarily offered support with regard to methodology and scientific approach. The support group consists of delegations of Dutch Stoma Care Association, the Dutch Association of Dieticians, Dutch Urological Association, Dutch Society of Dermatology and Venereology, Dutch Society of Surgery, the Dutch Association of Hepato-Gastroenterology Physicians and Hanny Cobussen-Boekhorst, specialist nurse in continence and urostomy. Dansac facilitated group meetings by providing meeting space. The professional organization did not receive any financial support for the development of this guideline.

Now that the first Dutch Guideline on Stoma Care has been published, we trust that this document will assist health-care providers in the Netherlands to provide stoma care according to the current vision.

This guideline is compiled according to start-to-end process a patient goes through when receiving a stoma. In evidence-based medicine, the final recommendation is made by using the information from three types of sources: research knowledge, practical knowledge (knowledge of the health-care professionals/experts) and the wishes and skills of the patient.

Therefore, the opinion of the patients and the method of patient approach are repeatedly described, evidence is sought to substantiate this. Additionally, organizational and financial aspects have also been taken into account.

The first chapter is an account of the methodology. Chapter two names and describes prevalence and definitions. The third chapter concerns counselling and education in all phases. Chapters four, five and six describe the entire process that the patient goes through: the preoperative phase, the postoperative phase, the discharge phase and the follow-up phase. In chapter seven the organization of stoma care in the Netherlands is described. Here recommendations are found on how to organize and facilitate stoma care in order for it to be carried out according to the recommendations in this guideline. The last chapter focuses on the way this guideline should be implemented and its evaluation.

Note to the reader:
Together with the Dutch Ostomy Association (NSV) it was decided to refer, as follows, to a person with a stoma. In the preoperative and postoperative clinical phase he will be referred to as "patient" and after discharge from the hospital as "ostomate".
To improve readability of this guideline, the patient is referred to as "he", the nurse as "she".

Recommendations

	Recommendation	Conclusion level
1	Work methodically and according to procedures to obtain the desired result within the limited time available with regard to providing important information about the stoma and teaching ostomy skills. Use a checklist.	3
2	Adapt counselling, education and training to the wishes, needs and abilities of the patient.	3
3	Provide the patient with all the necessary information to enable him to, should he so wish partake in the decision making process with regard to the diagnosis and choice of treatment.	3
4	Support the (potential) stoma patient by determining his coping style and applying an effective coping strategy.	3
5	Be aware of the impact that the construction of and living with a stoma has on the quality of the ostomate's life.	2
6	During counselling, education and training, the effects of the altered body image through the stoma on the patient should be considered.	4
7	Be aware of the impact that the construction of and living with a stoma has on the ostomate's sexual functioning.	2
8	Ask the stoma patient for permission to discuss the subject of sexuality. Then provide counselling, support or advice or refer him to other professionals.	3
9	Respect each other's cultures, beliefs and habits. Be familiar with the specific problems with respect to the stoma, which may arise due to lifestyle or instructions of other cultures and religions.	4
10	In case of emergency surgery, provide adjusted information, education and training as soon as the stoma patient is able to co-operate. Keep in mind that it requires more time than in the case of a planned operation.	4
11	Provide information oral and in writing and complement if necessary with multimedia. Adjust the use of various educational tools to the needs and possibilities of the stoma patient.	3
12	Offer the (potential) stoma patient the opportunity to participate in a support group.	3

	Recommendation	Conclusion level
13	Provide stoma information and counselling in the preoperative phase.	2
14	Provide the patient with information during the preoperative consultation with regard to receiving a stoma and the consequences for everyday life.	3
15	The spouse and/or relatives of the stoma patient should be involved in preoperative education.	3

16	Ensure that preoperative siting of the stoma becomes a standard procedure, which is always done in consultation with the patient. This has to be done with every patient who has to undergo surgery where a stoma will definitely or possibly be constructed.	2
17	When locating the stoma site, take into account positional issues, physical and patient-related considerations, and preferences of the patient and medical specialist.	2
18	In the case of an obese stomach, mark the stoma site, in consultation with the patient, above the umbilicus.	4
19	Discuss with the patient whether he wants to see, apply and/or remove different stoma appliances in the preoperative phase.	3

Postoperative phase and discharge phase; Chapter 5

	Recommendation	Conclusion level
20	Perform specific observations relating to the stoma immediately after surgery until the first 48 hours. These observations should be performed at least every eight hours.	4
21	Make sure that transparent stoma material is applied so that postoperative stoma observations can be performed properly.	4
22	Provide active support or co-ordinate self-care teaching. Adapt the pace of teaching self-care to each individual stoma patient.	4
23	In consultation with the stoma patient, the spouse and/or relatives should be involved in the process of learning to take care of the stoma.	3
24	In the discharge phase, in consultation with the stoma patient, all aspects that need to be taken care of before being discharged from hospital, should be checked systematically.	3
25	Ensure that the stoma care nurse is in charge of the stoma care in the postoperative phase.	3
26	Provide the stoma patient with general recommendations on healthy eating.	4
27	Ensure that the ileostomy patient, prior to discharge from the hospital, is given information by a dietician on fluid intake, nutrition and consumption of extra salt.	4
28	Ensure that the urostomy patient receives adequate advice on required fluid intake, to achieve pale yellow or straw coloured urine.	4
29	Advise the urostomy patient about the remedial benefits of cranberry juice or capsules in the event of skin- or leakage problems or (symptomatic) urinary tract infections.	3
30	Use clear, validated descriptions of the complications. Work from these valid definitions to further uniformity in nursing interventions.	3
31	Use a measuring instrument for describing and diagnosing peristomal skin disorders.	4
32	Ensure the stoma patient is aware of the symptoms related to the various potential complications or problems.	3

33	Attempt to use a stoma appliance that best suits the characteristics of the stoma, and the characteristics and personal preferences of the stoma patient.	3
34	Check regularly during three months after surgery, in consultation with the stoma patient, whether the opening of the skin barrier still fits the stoma. If necessary, adjust the stoma appliance.	4
35	Inform the stoma patient about the disposal of used stoma appliances.	4
36	In the event of complications or problems, inform the stoma patient whether a stoma care aid is indicated and, if needed and in consultation with the stoma patient, make a choice from the accessories available.	4

Aftercare phase; Chapter 6

	Recommendation	Conclusion level
37	Ensure that, in consultation with the ostomate, follow-up check-ups by the stoma care nurse take place.	3
38	Schedule the check-ups at the stoma care nurse and physician simultaneously.	3
39	Advise the ostomate to meet with the stoma care nurse for follow-up visits, starting within two weeks after discharge from hospital, thereafter every six weeks for the following three months and then after six months.	3
40	Advise the ostomate to visit the stoma care nurse once a year, from the second year after surgery onwards, for a general stoma check-up. Adjust the care to the individual ostomate and if necessary, adjust appointment-frequency.	3
41	Discuss the home situation with the ostomate to determine whether home-support and -counselling is needed to help deal with the day-to day situation. It may concern practical as well as psychosocial assistance.	3
42	Ensure that, in consultation with the ostomate, a complete transfer is done, with the aim of guaranteeing continuity of expert stoma care.	3
43	Provide the ostomate with information about the added value of follow-up visits with regard to the prevention and incidence of stomal and peristomal problems.	3
44	Ensure as a stoma care nurse, to have knowledge of all available stoma accessories and aids and their applicability.	4
45	In the event of complications or other problems, inform the ostomate about other available stoma accessories. In consultation with the ostomate, supported by the expertise of the stoma care nurse, make a selection from the available materials.	4
46	After consultation with the physician, inform the ostomate about the possibility of irrigation. Ensure that the instruction is done by the stoma care nurse. The amount of water used during, the frequency of, and the time required for flushing, differs for each person.	3
47	Advise to use a cone rather than a catheter for irrigation.	4

48	Advise the ostomate to stay under supervision of a stoma care nurse during pregnancy, because adjustments of the stoma appliance and additional counselling may be needed.	4
49	If necessary, contact the midwife or obstetrician.	4
50	For obese ostomates additional information should be provided and extra check-ups are required due to the increased risk of physical problems and complications.	3
51	Involve relatives of obese patients since there is a chance the obese patient will require more assistance due to the increased risk of physical problems and complications.	4

Organizing stoma care; Chapter 7

	Recommendation	Conclusion level
52	Adjust the level of job-competence to the complexity of the care. Uncomplicated stoma care can be executed from level three IG. In the case of abnormal situations or complications a level four or five nurse should be allocated to the patient.	4
53	Refer the ostomate to the stoma care nurse in the event of complications.	4
54	Ensure that there are sufficient trained nurses available to achieve good care outcomes.	2
55	Ensure that the stoma care nurse acts as a case manager, in order to promote multidisciplinary co-operation between all the care professionals involved.	4
56	Ensure that a stoma care nurse is employed in each institution where stoma care is offered. These institutions should facilitate the stoma care nurses.	3
57	Make sure that the ostomate has access to a stoma care nurse.	2
58	Promote the continuity of stoma care in the home situation by employing a stoma care nurse in the outpatient setting.	4
59	Ensure as a stoma care nurse to get sufficient training and practical experience and stay well informed on developments within the field of ostomy care.	4
60	Ensure as a stoma care nurse registration in the V&VN quality register and the subregister of ostomy care.	4

Chapter 1 Methodology

This chapter describes how the guideline came into being. The public script of the VIKC (Association of Comprehensive Cancer Centres, the Dutch national association of eight comprehensive cancer centres in the Netherlands) was used as starting point. Then a script was developed in which the process of development, implementation and evaluation of the guideline is described. For the realization of this guideline, the EBRO (evidence-based guideline development) method of the CBO was used.

The starting point for this guideline is the analysis of problem areas experienced in stoma care. This analysis was performed from different points of view (nurses, patients and organizational perspective), and different methods were used:
a. A survey filled out by stoma care nurses during an association meeting (March 2009). Questionnaires were distributed and collected later on the same day. 105 valid questionnaires were used for analysis.
b. Work protocol comparison. Ten protocols on colostomy care were obtained from intramural end extramural health-care facilities throughout the Netherlands.
c. An analysis of "De kwaliteit van de stomazorg in patiëntenperspectief. Een set van kwaliteitscriteria" (The quality of ostomy care in perspective. A set of quality criteria) (Nederlandse Stomavereniging, 2008).
The results from these three analyses showed many similarities: the shift of stoma care to a lower level care provider, lack of broad (basic) knowledge, lack of clarity and gaps in the continuity of care (intramural/extramural). In addition, the Dutch Stoma Care Association also put forward problem areas: the manner in which, and the groups to whom the stoma care nurse gives information such as other health-care providers involved in stoma care, the ostomate's freedom to choose stoma accessories and, that in counselling, alternative treatment options with pros and cons need to be mentioned.

Starting out from the analysis of problem areas, the following questions were formulated:
• Definition stomata: How is a stoma defined? (Permanent, temporary, adult).
• How often do the various stomata occur (colo-ileo-uro); what is the incidence and prevalence?
• What is considered to be standard stoma care in the preoperative phase?
• Preoperative information and education: What is understood by appropriate patient information/education.?
• What is considered to be standard postoperative phase stoma care?
• Postoperative information and education: What is understood by appropriate patient information/education?
• Complications of stoma construction in the postoperative stage/discharge phase. Definitions, prevention, recognition, identification and treatment.
• Choice of postoperative appliances: When to use which appliance?
• What is considered to be standard aftercare phase stoma care?
• Aftercare information and education: What is understood by appropriate patient information/education?

- Complications of stoma construction in the aftercare phase. Definitions, prevention, recognition, identification and treatment.
- Choice of appliances in the aftercare phase: When to use which appliance?
- Which care provider performs which care and when; what level of expertise is required?
- Which continuity of care is desirable?
- What medical disciplines are involved in stoma care?
- Other aspects.

With these questions as starting point, search terms were formulated. Using these terms, a search was conducted in, amongst others, PubMed, Cinahl and Cochrane. Books, magazines and guidelines from other countries were also consulted for information. In order to guarantee completeness, these terms were again used to search databases. The search terms that were used can be found in Appendix III.

120 different search terms were used in various combinations, with different limits. Limits agreed upon were: Humans, English, Dutch, All Adult: 19 + years, published in the last 10 years. Excluding topics were: gastrostomy, tracheostomy and nephrostomy.

In addition, reference lists in the publications found and consulted were checked for possible titles missed in the initial search. This effort yielded dozens more titles. The above-mentioned agreed limits were not applied on these titles.

Throughout the whole process, 323 titles of research articles, opinion pieces, books and other publications were eventually found. Many articles (211) were excluded. The most common reasons for exclusion were: publication date (more recent publications on the same subject available), general case description on either one patient, a small group of patients, or the situation was not representative for the Netherlands. Some publications were not available at all or not available in either English or Dutch (only an abstract in English). Several articles were rejected because the approach to the subject was too medical or did not answer the questions. After exclusion 112 usable publications remained.

After having determined whether the usable publication was a work of research or an opinion piece the studies were reviewed with help of the existing EBRO forms, as recommended by the CBO (www.cbo.nl/thema/Richtlijnen/). Following this assessment, each study was categorized based on the level of evidence and according to classification; refer to table 1 and 2. In addition to this, the form "evaluate nursing research" (Hunink, 1996) was used for comparative nursing research.

	Intervention	Diagnostic accuracy study	Damage or side effects, etiology, prognosis *
A1	Systematic review of at least two independently conducted A2 level studies		
A2	High standard, sufficiently sized, randomized, double-blind, comparative, clinical studies	Study relative to a referenced test ('golden standard') with predefined cut-off values and independent assessment of the results of test and golden standard, on a sufficiently large series of consecutive patients, all of them having had the index and reference test	Prospective cohort study of sufficient size and follow-up, where 'confounding' was adequately controlled and selective follow-up was sufficiently excluded.
B	Comparative study, but not including all the features listed under A2 (this includes patient-control studies, cohort studies)	Study relative to a referenced test, but not with all the features listed under A2	Prospective cohort study, but not including all the features listed under A2 or retrospective cohort or patient-control study
C	Non-comparative study		
D	Expert opinion		

Table 1. Classification of methodological quality of individual studies

Level	Study
+ +	Credible meta-synthesis (synonyms: meta-ethnography, qualitative meta - analysis, meta-study) of qualitative studies
+	Credible study
+/-	Study with questionable credibility.
-	Study with low credibility.

Table 2. Gradation of qualitative research

In this search phase, three existing guidelines on stoma care were found and assessed using the AGREE (Appraisal of Guidelines for Research and Evaluation), a tool for assessing guidelines (www.cbo.nl/thema/Richtlijnen/Partnerships/AGREE/). These three guidelines are "Ostomy care and management" by the Registered Nurses' Association of Ontario (RNAO, Canada), "Incontinent urostomy" written by EAUN (European association of urology nurses) and "Management of the patient with a fecal ostomy: best practice guidelines for clinicians" by the Wound Ostomy and Continence Nurses Society (WOCN, United States). All three guidelines are considered usable under conditions or in the event of changes. In practice this means that parts of these guidelines are useful: sometimes the contents, sometimes the way the guideline is classified or how the information is presented. Additionally, the existing "Guideline on stoma care, subtopic: determining the stoma site preoperatively "(May, 2006) by the V&VN Department of Stoma Care Nurses, was reviewed, updated and subsequently included in this guideline. After having evaluated the various sources on quality and contents, the working group then proceeded to search abovementioned documents and publications for answers to the clinical questions. Although the guideline is organized based on the process the stoma patient follows, it sometimes proved to be more logical to cluster a number of questions and answer them all together. When this is the case, it is mentioned. Also, certain topics are addressed more than once, for example attention to spouse and relatives. However, this is always done in context of the specific phase under discussion.

Finally, a level of evidence is mentioned by each recommendation. The conclusions' level of evidence is based on the evidence which forms the underlying basis for the conclusion: refer to table 3.

In relation to the level of evidence the corresponding recommendation is formulated. The manner of formulating each recommendation is directly related to the strength of the evidence. However, the level of evidence related to each individual recommendation is also mentioned.

	Conclusion based on
1	Study of level A1 or at least 2 independent studies of level A2
2	1 study of level A2 or at least 2 independent studies of level B
3	1 study of level B or C
4	Opinion of experts

Table 3. Level of evidence of the conclusion

Chapter 2 Definition, prevalence and indications

This chapter focuses on definitions. The most commonly used terms are defined, prevalence is described, as well as reasons why a stoma would be necessary.

This chapter provides answers to three questions:

How does one define a stoma? (permanent, temporary, adults)

How often do various stomata occur? (colo-ileo-uro)

What is the incidence and prevalence?

2.1. Definition

The working group defines a stoma as: an artificial, surgically constructed opening which connects a portion of the body cavity to the outside environment.

This guideline applies to "incontinent" stomata (colostomy, ileostomy, urostomy) in adults. In Appendix IV as many definitions and terms as possible, associated with the stoma, are described.

2.2. Incidence and prevalence

No reliable statistics on the incidence and prevalence of people with a stoma are known. Despite the fact that various sources have been checked (e.g. RIVM, health insurers, hospitals, DICA/DSCA) no absolute figures are available. This can be explained by the fact that a stoma is not defined as a disease or a condition. The diseases or conditions where a stoma usually is required are registered as such, but whether or not a stoma was constructed, is not recorded separately. Therefore we have to be content with estimates.

The Ostomy Platform is a network which unites the different parties in the Netherlands involved in ostomy care (patient associations, professional associations, manufacturers, suppliers). This platform estimates that there are approximately 32,000 ostomates in the Netherlands. In addition, it is estimated that 7,000 new stomata are constructed each year. There is no information available on the ratio between permanent and temporary stomata.

In foreign literature, no reliable figures regarding number of ostomates could be found. The various publications also presented varying data. The articles and the three foreign guidelines all state the numbers to be estimates.

2.3. Indications

There are many different reasons for the necessity of a stoma. Summarised, the most common reasons why a stoma is constructed is cancer (colon carcinoma, bladder carcinoma), inflammatory bowel disease (Crohn's disease and Colitis ulcerosa), incontinence and neurological disorders.

In Appendix V the different indications are listed in alphabetical order for each type of stoma.

Chapter 3 Information and education in stoma care

A question from the analysis of problem areas, information and education, that will be discussed in this chapter is: What is understood by appropriate patient information/education?
This question returns in all the phases but will be discussed and answered in this chapter. In answering this question, important aspects concerning counselling and education were examined. The contents of the counselling, however, will be discussed in the following chapters.

3.1. Definitions
During the different phases (preoperative, postoperative clinical and aftercare) the patient can be provided with counselling, information, education and training.
These concepts easily overlap.
Counselling is "giving information through communication, allowing an interested person to come to a well-balanced decision and forming opinions in a concrete situation". (translation from www.woorden-boek.nl/woord/voorlichting dd. 4-2-12)
Information is "data that increases knowledge". (translation from www.woorden.org/woord/informatie dd. 10-11-11)
Education is "the conscious and deliberate creation of conditions and organization of activities and learning for some time, to increase knowledge and insight". (translation from www.mijnwoordenboek.nl/vertaal/NL/NL/educatie dd. 10-11-11)
Training is "learning, improving or changing social, cognitive and psycho-motor skills". (translation from www.mijnwoordenboek.nl/vertaal/NL/NL/training dd. 10-11-11).

3.2. Providing information
The stoma care nurse is aware of the fact that every individual comprehends and understands information in his own way. O'Shea (2001) indicates that providing information to a stoma patient is based on principles of adult education. In addition, the willingness, ability and need of the patient to learn is also assessed.
The stoma care nurse adapts to the individual patient, for example, geriatric patients, patients with disabilities, with cognitive impairment, with reading difficulties or with potential cultural barriers that have to be overcome. O 'Shea points out that counselling takes place both planned and incidental. Scheduled or planned counselling is based on pre-established goals. Incidental counselling happens whenever the patient has a question which needs to be answered, for instance during stoma care. In this way counselling can even be given regarding lifestyle, without this being emphasized too much.
Regarding counselling, education and training, the patient and the nurse have expectations towards each other. The patient assumes that the nurse is educated, competent and willing to share information. The nurse on the other hand, expects from the patient a willingness to learn and to have an open-mind with regard to the necessary changes in his lifestyle.
According to Brown and Randle (2005) the sharing of information should be systematically and according to a pre-determined procedure. This helps to provide the necessary information within the time available. Furthermore, the stoma care nurse should be aware that patients may respond in different ways and that the response may also change during the process. To ensure

co-operation between patient and nurse, it is important that they both have a feeling of being allies and that the nurse adjusts to the level of understanding of the patient and his relatives. Readding (2005) states that from the very first contact with the patient, the nurse has to focus on how the patient will continue with his life after surgery.

Based on the review of the literature, O 'Connor (2005) describes the appropriate way to educate the ostomate. This education is simultaneously aimed at teaching self-care. It explores the methods best utilized by the stoma care nurse in teaching stoma care in the pre- and postoperative phases. Proper organization, supported by sound teaching principles, curriculae and the help of a checklist are all of importance, so that no vital aspects are forgotten. There is dialogue with the patient and his willingness and ability to learn is engaged. Research shows that patients are able to deal better with the stoma, if they are encouraged to learn stoma management straightaway. Therefore, this should commence in the preoperative phase and continue till the postoperative phase. A good transfer when discharged from hospital, with continuation of the learning process after discharge, promotes successful rehabilitation. O'Connor advocates that the stoma patient should only be discharged from hospital after having shown that he disposes of enough skills to empty and change a stoma bag.

Recommendation 1: (as concluded from the abovementioned)
Work methodically and according to procedures to obtain the desired result within the limited time available with regard to providing important information about the stoma and teaching ostomy skills. Use a checklist (for example Appendix VI).

Recommendation 2: (as concluded from the abovementioned)
Adapt counselling, education and training to the wishes, needs and abilities of the patient.

Conclusion level 3	
level	Author title
B	Brown, H. & Randle, J. (2005). Living with a stoma: a review of the literature. *Journal of clinical nursing, 14,* 74-81.
D	O'Connor, G. (2005). Teaching stoma-management skills: the importance of self-care. *British journal of nursing, 14(4),* 320-324.
D	O' Shea, H.S. (2001). Teaching the adult ostomy patient. *Journal of wound ostomy continence nursing, 28(1),* 47-54.
D	Readding, L.A. (2005). Hospital to home, smoothing the journey for the new ostomist. *British journal of nursing, 14(16),* 16-20.

3.3. Shared decision-making

Shared decision-making aims to involve the patient in the care and in decision-making as far as diagnosis and treatment are concerned. This can have an encouraging effect on the co-operation between patient and care provider.

Research shows that proper organizing and support of this process can be of great help to patients. They are better informed, more aware of the advantages and disadvantages of certain choices and often feel more content and are less doubtful about their decision (www.zelfmanagement.com/thema-s/shared-decision-making/, dd. 19.11.11).

Also Persson et al (2005b) describe that patients need sufficient information to be able to make good decisions. If the information is insufficient, people cannot adequately participate in the process, which can lead to discontentment. The stoma care nurse should therefore always be ready and willing to share information. Persson states that the extent to which the patient is involved in the decision-making process in the preoperative phase regarding the treatment, is indicative to his adaptability. The role of the patient changes from a passive to a more active role. According to Persson self-care should be provided, where possible, in close co-operation with the patient, taking into account his needs and wishes. She states that previous studies emphasize the importance of the involvement of the patient with regard to all aspects of his disease and the possibility to express his feelings. She also maintains that people who receive preoperative education are more content when they are actively involved in decision-making during the disease.

O 'Shea (2001) assumes that on-going professional training is essential to the professional nurse to ensure that the patient has sufficient knowledge, enabling him to give consent for treatment and that he is aware of the normal postoperative procedures.

Recommendation 3: (as concluded from the abovementioned)
Provide the patient with all the necessary information to enable him to, should he so wish partake in the decision making process with regard to the diagnosis and choice of treatment.

Conclusion level 3	
level	Author title
C	Persson, E., Gustavsson, B., Hellström, A.L., Lappas, G., Hultén, L. (2005 b). Ostomy patients' perceptions of quality of care. *Journal of advanced nursing, 49(1),* 51-58.
D	O' Shea, H.S. (2001). Teaching the adult ostomy patient. *Journal of wound ostomy continence nursing, 28(1),* 47-54

3.4. Coping

With regard to the counselling, education and training of the (potential) stoma patient, the stoma care nurse should consider the situation of the patient. At this stage a stoma is often not the only thing the patient has to deal with, the disease itself also calls for attention and processing. The situation could be uncertain because the progress of the disease and the required treatment may not yet be clear. It is therefore important to take account of the coping styles of the patient.

Potter (2000) describes that stoma care nurses can have a positive impact on the adaptions that are needed. This can be achieved by providing accurate information, expert care, supportive education, assisting in setting realistic goals and to determine what coping strategies the patient uses.

Simmons et al (2007) conducted descriptive studies on the acceptance of the stoma and adaptions in daily life and the descriptive study of Tseng et al (2004) relates to stress factors in outpatients with a colostomy. Both claim that good stoma care also include strategies which encourage patients to accept the stoma and to take up their social activities again. Stoma care nurses must encourage patients to resume their normal daily life.

The Gouveia Santos et al (2006) conducted a descriptive research on using coping strategies and quality of life. The conclusion was that there is a difference in coping strategies between people with a temporary stoma and those with a permanent stoma. Patients with a temporary stoma more often use a strategy of avoidance, whilst those with a permanent stoma apply a strategy of active problem solving.

In a study by Reynaud and Meeker (2002) a questionnaire was completed by geriatrics (aged 50-84 years) to investigate coping styles. Independent and optimistic styles are most commonly used as an effective coping style by people with a stoma. This indicates that a positive and independent way of life, generally speaking, prevails over dependence on others in dealing with the stoma as a "stress factor". Part of the role of the stoma care nurse is to find out which concerns or anxieties the stoma patient is experiencing. Consequently the stoma care nurse can help the patient identify a coping style and support him the implementation of an effective coping strategy. Preoperative and postoperative education, guidance and sustained support given by the stoma care nurse, helps the patient to deal with stress more effectively.

Recommendation 4: (as concluded from the abovementioned)
Support the (potential) stoma patient by determining his coping style and applying an effective coping strategy.

Conclusion level 3	
level	**Author title**
C	Simmons, K.L., Smith, J.A., Bobb, K.A. & Liles, L.L.M. (2007). Adjustment to colostomy: stoma acceptance, stoma care self-efficacy and interpersonal relationships. *Journal of Advanced Nursing, 60(6)*, 627-635.
C	Tseng, H.C., Wang, H.H., Hsu, Y.Y. & Weng, W.C. (2004). Factors related to stress in outpatients with permanent colostomies. *Kaohsiung J. Med. Sci., 20(2)*, 70-77.
C	Reynaud, S.N. & Meeker, B.J. (2002). Coping styles of older adults with ostomies. *Journal of gerontological nursing, 28(5),* 30 -36.
++	De Gouveia Santos, V.L.C., Chaves, E.C. & Kimura, M. (2006). Quality of life and coping of persons with temporary and permanent stomas. *Journal of Wound Ostomy Continence Nursing, 33(5),* 503-509.
D	Potter, K.L. (2000). Surgical oncology of the pelvis: ostomy planning and management. *Journal of Surgical oncology, 73,* 237-242.

3.5. Quality of life, body image, sexuality
The influence of the stoma on sexuality and quality of life is addressed in several studies. In some studies the issue of changing body image was included.

3.5.1. Influence of the stoma on quality of life
Cotrim and Pereira (2008) examined the impact of colorectal cancer on patients and their families. The follow-up period was six to eight months after surgery. One of the results from this study was that people with a stoma indicated that they have a lesser overall quality of life than those without a stoma.

Ross et al (2006) carried out research into quality of life of people with and without a stoma after colorectal cancer, during a period of 24 months after surgery. This study also showed that people with a stoma indicate a lesser quality of life than those without a stoma. An additional result from this research is that when people are to receive a stoma at a later stage (because of complications), they experience a worsening of quality of life.

The report of the Dutch Ostomy Association "The influence of the stoma on daily life" (2009b) states that 34 percent of people feel that the stoma has reduced their quality of life. This shows that there is a link between the evaluation of quality of life and the perceived health. There is also a link between the reason for a stoma and the perceived quality of life: more people with bladder cancer and colon cancer indicate that the quality of life has deteriorated compared to people with Crohn's disease or Colitis ulcerosa.

Recommendation 5: (as concluded from the abovementioned).
Be aware of the impact that the construction of and living with a stoma has on the quality of the ostomate's life.

Conclusion Level 2	
level	Author title
B	Cotrim, H. & Pereira, G. (2008). Impact of colorectal cancer on patient and family: implications for care. European journal of oncology nursing, 12, 217- 226.
B	Ross, L., Abild-Nielsen, A.G., Thomsen, B.L., Karlsen, R.V., Boesen, E.H. & Johansen, C. (2006). Quality of life of Danish colorectal cancer patients with and without a stoma. *Support Care Cancer, 15(5),* 505-513.
C	Nederlandse Stomavereniging (2009b). *De invloed van de stoma op het dagelijks leven. Onderzoeksverslag in opdracht van de NSV.* Amsterdam: Newcom Research & Consultancy B.V. Kapteijns, A. & Buitinga, S.

3.5.2. Changing body image
Thorpe et al (2009) reviewed qualitative studies addressing the impact of the stoma on patients' altered body image. In these studies, three broad themes were identified: the loss of bodily wholeness (see definitions in Appendix IV), the awareness of a damaged body and disturbed confidence in the altered body. The conclusion of this review is that nurses must be aware of the impact of an altered body image caused by the stoma and the consequences for self-image. Black (2004) indicates that stoma care nurses must be aware of the process that a patient with altered body image goes through. The phases in this process range from denial and avoidance to acceptance.

Recommendation 6: (as concluded from the abovementioned)
During counselling, education and training, the effects of the altered body image through the stoma on the patient should be considered.

Conclusion Level 4	
level	Author title
++	Thorpe, G., McArthur, M. & Richardson, B. (2009). Bodily change following faecal stoma formation: qualitative interpretive synthesis. *Journal of Advanced Nursing, Review Paper, 65(9),* 1778 -1789.
D	Black, PK (2004). Psychological, sexual and cultural issues for patients with a stoma. *British journal of nursing, 13(12),* 692-697.

3.5.3. Influence of stoma on sexuality

Brown and Randle (2005) describe that several studies show that patients experienced a decline in sexual attractiveness since receiving a stoma.

A study by Kilic et al (2007) among people with a permanent stoma in Turkey revealed that women with a stoma experience more problems related to sexuality than women without a stoma. This is explained by the physiological changes after surgery.

Black (2004) indicates that through surgery and/or radiation in the pelvic area (in bladder and colorectal surgery) the tissue as well as the vascular- and nerve supply is damaged to such an extent that a loss of function occurs.

Pieper and Mikols (1996) also indicate that people with a stoma experience sexual problems and that this should be discussed with the stoma patients and their spouses.

Recommendation 7: (as concluded from the abovementioned).
Be aware of the impact that the construction of and living with a stoma has on the ostomate's sexual functioning.

Conclusion Level 2	
level	Author title
B	Brown, H. & Randle, J. (2005). Living with a stoma: a review of the literature. Journal of clinical nursing, 14, 74-81.
B	Kilic, E., Taycan, O., Belli, A.K. & Özmen, M. (2007). The effect of permanent ostomy on body image, self-esteem, marital adjustment, and sexual functioning. *Turkish Journal of Psychiatry, 18(4)*, 1-8.
C	Pieper, B. & Mikols, C. (1996). Predischarge and postdischarge concerns of persons with an ostomy. Journal of wound ostomy continence nursing, 23(2), 105-109.
D	Black, P.K. (2004). Psychological, sexual and cultural issues for patients with a stoma. British journal of nursing, 13(12), 692-697.

3.5.4. Discussing the subject of sexuality

The European "incontinent urostomy" guideline (EAUN, 2009) mentions that the construction of a stoma in both men and women can lead to problematic sexual functioning. Often however, much can be achieved with the help of medication and aids. In cases where sexual dis-functioning as a result of the operation can be expected, the patients should be informed preoperatively about the consequences and possible solutions for the future. During the postoperative counselling these subjects should be addressed repeatedly.

Persson et al (2005 a) describe that both patient and spouse are often dissatisfied about the possibilities, during consultations, to discuss sexual consequences of stoma construction surgery with the stoma care nurse.

Persson et al (2005 b) stresses that the responsibility of discussing sexuality lies with the stoma care nurse.

Black (2004) too advocates that the subject of sexuality should be discussed by the stoma care nurse, that it should be included in basic care. According to Black, many nurses find it difficult to have an open discussion about sexuality. The stoma care nurse should be knowledgeable of the impact of the operation on sexuality. She should be aware of the different possibilities of treatment and also understand when her own competences and job description come into play.

With sufficient knowledge and skills, the stoma care nurse can provide the ostomate as well as the spouse with sound information, be supportive and offer advice on the possibilities of treatment and/or referral to the specialised help of an urologist or sexologist (Black, 2004). Junkin and Beitz (2005) indicate that sexuality as a topic has to be part of the total care. The stoma care nurse can make use of the PLISSIT model to discuss sexuality. PLISSIT is a conversation model and the letters form an anagram for Permission, Low threshold Information, Specific Suggestions, Intensive Therapy.

Recommendation 8: (as concluded from the above mentioned).
Ask the stoma patient for permission to discuss the subject of sexuality. Then provide counselling, support or advice or refer him to other professionals.

Conclusion Level 3	
level	Author title
C	Persson, E., Gustavsson, B., Hellström, A.L., Fridstedt, G., Lappas, G., Hultén, L. (2005 a). Information to the relatives of people with ostomies. *Journal of wound ostomy continence nursing, 32(4)*, 238-245.
C	Persson, E., Gustavsson, B., Hellström, A.L., Lappas, G., Hultén, L. (2005 b). Ostomy patients' perceptions of quality of care. *Journal of advanced nursing, 49(1)*, 51-58.
D	Black, P.K. (2004). Psychological, sexual and cultural issues for patients with a stoma. British journal of nursing, 13(12), 692-697.
D	Junkin, J. & Beitz, J. (2005). Sexuality and the person with a stoma: Impliciations for comprehensive WOC nursing practice. *Journal of wound ostomy continence nursing, 32(2)*, 121-128.
AGREE	European Association of Urology Nurses (2009). *Good practice in health care: incontinent urstomy.* European Association of Urology Nurses Geng, V., Cobussen, H., Fillingham, S., Holroyd, S., Kiesbye, B. & Vahr, S.

3.6. Cultural and religious aspects

Both EAUN (2009) and Black (2004) report that the stoma care nurse must be well aware of the influence of different cultures and religions. In our modern multicultural society, self-care workers should be respectful to each individual's cultural background, religion and customs. Religion and culture can be the reason for a patient to make different choices in interventions and treatment, which can prove to be even more difficult due to possible language barriers. In the event of language problems, an interpreter can be of help and an imam may be helpful for Muslim patients. Attention has to be given to the various nutritional aspects regarding religion or culture, such as vegetarian food or fasting (Ramadan) (EAUN 2009, Black, 2004). For specific questions about nutrition, patients can also be referred to a dietician

Recommendation 9: (as concluded from the abovementioned)
Respect each other's cultures, beliefs and habits. Be familiar with the specific problems with respect to the stoma, which may arise due to lifestyle or instructions of other cultures and religions.

Conclusion Level 4	
level	Author title
AGREE	European Association of Urology Nurses (2009). *Good practice in health care: incontinent urstomy.* European Association of Urology Nurses Geng, V., Cobussen, H., Fillingham, S., Holroyd, S., Kiesbye, B. & Vahr, S.
D	Black, PK (2004). Psychological, sexual and cultural issues for patients with a stoma. British journal of nursing, 13(12), 692-697.

3.7. Emergency surgery guidance

When a patient urgently needs surgery it is usually not possible to provide counselling before the operation. However, it should explicitly be strived after to at least decide on the location of the stoma (see also Section 4.2.B.). Vujnovich (2009) recommends that dosed information should be given two or three days after the operation. She indicates that these patients may experience more stress and tension because of the stoma than people who have had preoperative information. With counselling in the postoperative phase it should be taken into account that the patient may need more time to internalize the information, it may also take longer before adapting to life with a stoma.

Even Potter (2000) indicates that in the event of emergency surgery, or if the stoma had to be constructed unexpectedly, more time is needed postoperatively for information sharing and education. The relationship between the patient and the stoma care nurse still needs to be established while the patient suffers postoperative pain and other discomfort.

The above is in accordance with the contents of Appendix VI about preoperative information.

Recommendation 10: (as concluded from the abovementioned)

In case of emergency surgery, provide adjusted information, education and training as soon as the stoma patient is able to co-operate. Keep in mind that it requires more time than in the case of a planned operation.

Conclusion Level 4	
level	Author title
D	Vujnovich, A. (2008) Pre and post- operative assessment of patients with a stoma. *Nursing standard, 22(19), 50-56.*
D	Potter, K.L. (2000). Surgical oncology of the pelvis: ostomy planning and management. *Journal of Surgical oncology, 73, 237-242.*

3.8. Information, tools and resources

Besides the oral information being shared during a consultation, there are many other ways of exchanging information.

In the report "Kwaliteit en organisatie van stomazorg" (Quality and organization of the stoma care) (NSV, 2009 c) sixteen percent of respondents indicated that they received insufficient written information, in spite of the fact that various studies have been clear on the value of written information. It enables the patient to reread the information and it also provides information for relatives and other people close to the patient (Burch, 2008).

O'Connor (2005), O'Shea (2001) as well as Vujnovich (2007) suggest the use of appropriate written brochures and drawings during the preoperative counselling. Erwin-Toth (2006) indicates that drawings, photographs, DVD's or other images can support the oral and written information. Potter (2000) recommends using drawings to explain the anatomy of the colon, which part of the intestine is to be removed or what change will take place.

Lo et al (2009) studied the effect of the use of multimedia in preoperative counselling. When a patient had a consultation with a stoma care nurse in combination with watching an informative film, it resulted in cost reduction. In the postoperative phase, the self-care aspect was grasped faster.

In the preoperative consultation the patient may also be advised to read up on the subject on informative, relevant websites.

Vujnovic (2008) recommends offering the possibility of getting in touch with a support group. These patient groups can offer oral or written, non-medical advice about living with a stoma. During counselling in the preoperative phase, the stoma care nurse can ask whether the patient would appreciate joining a support group and if so, the contact person can be informed.

Recommendation 11: (as concluded from the abovementioned)
Provide information oral and in writing and complement if necessary with multimedia. Adjust the use of various educational tools to the needs and possibilities of the stoma patient.

Recommendation 12: (as concluded from the abovementioned)
Offer the (potential) stoma patient the opportunity to participate in a support group.

Conclusion Level 3	
level	**Author title**
B	Lo, S.F., Wang, Y.T., Hsu, M.Y., Chang S.C. & Hayter, M. (2009). A cost-effectiveness analysis of a multimedia learning education program for stoma patients. *Journal of Clinical Nursing, Epup: 4,* 1-11.
C	Nederlandse Stomavereniging (2009c). *Kwaliteit en organisatie van stomazorg. Onderzoeksverslag in opdracht van de NSV .* Amsterdam: Newcom Research & Consultancy B.V. Kapteijns, A. & Buitinga, S.
D	Burch, J. (2008). Stomacare. *John Wiley & Sons, Chichester* ISBN 978-0-470-03177-3
D	O'Connor, G., (2005). Teaching stoma-management skills: the importance of selfcare. *British journal of nursing, 14(4),* 320-324.
D	O' Shea, H.S. (2001). Teaching the adult ostomy patient. *Journal of wound ostomy continence nursing, 28(1),* 47-54.
D	Vujnovich, A. (2008) Pre and post- operative assessment of patients with a stoma. *Nursing standard, 22(19),* 50-56.
D	Erwin-Toth, P., (2006). Ostomy care and rehabilitation in colorectal cancer. *Seminars in oncology nursing, 22(3),* 174-177.
D	Potter, K.L. (2000). Surgical oncology of the pelvis: ostomy planning and management. *Journal of Surgical oncology, 73,* 237-242.

	Recommendation	Conclusion level
1	Work methodically and according to procedures to obtain the desired result within the limited time available with regard to providing important information about the stoma and teaching ostomy skills. Use a checklist.	3
2	Adapt counselling, education and training to the wishes, needs and abilities of the patient.	3
3	Provide the patient with all the necessary information to enable him to, should he so wish partake in the decision making process with regard to the diagnosis and choice of treatment.	3
4	Support the (potential) stoma patient by determining his coping style and applying an effective coping strategy.	3
5	Be aware of the impact that the construction of and living with a stoma has on the quality of the ostomate's life.	2
6	During counselling, education and training, the effects of the altered body image through the stoma on the patient should be considered.	4
7	Be aware of the impact that the construction of and living with a stoma has on the ostomate's sexual functioning.	2
8	Ask the stoma patient for permission to discuss the subject of sexuality. Then provide counselling, support or advice or refer him to other professionals.	3
9	Respect each other's cultures, beliefs and habits. Be familiar with the specific problems with respect to the stoma, which may arise due to lifestyle or instructions of other cultures and religions.	4
10	In case of emergency surgery, provide adjusted information, education and training as soon as the stoma patient is able to co-operate. Keep in mind that it requires more time than in the case of a planned operation.	4
11	Provide information oral and in writing and complement if necessary with multimedia. Adjust the use of various educational tools to the needs and possibilities of the stoma patient.	3
12	Offer the (potential) stoma patient the opportunity to participate in a support group.	3

Chapter 4 Preoperative phase

This chapter answers the following question: What is understood by standard stoma care in the preoperative phase and what requirements should be met?

4.1. Definition
The working group has defined this phase as the phase prior to surgery where a stoma might possibly be constructed. This usually happens on an outpatient basis, but can also take place in a clinical setting.

4.2. Standard stoma care in the preoperative phase
Stoma care in the preoperative phase comprises three elements: preoperative counselling, establishing stoma location and providing opportunity to wear and practice with stoma appliances.
Each of these three elements will be described.
In the event of emergency surgery every situation will be evaluated individually in order to assess what can be carried out preoperatively. Counselling and information will have to be adapted postoperatively.

4.2.A. Preoperative counselling
The goal of preoperative counselling is that the future ostomate understands the concept of a stoma and is aware of the consequences of having a stoma. The potential ostomate receives adequate information and education about the surgery and the consequences. (Adequately means 'suitable for the intended purpose'). Fioravanti (1988) argues that "Adequate information before surgery and during hospitalization, as a necessary component of patient care and a very important element in establishing the optimal functional and psychological recovery of patients with a stoma", has been proven.
The importance of raising awareness in the preoperative phase has been shown in various studies.
Research from Millan (2009) shows that preoperative counselling and establishing the location is essential for the acceptance of the stoma and prevention of complications. Patients who had a preoperative consultation with a stoma care nurse suffered significant less complications and anxiety than patients who had not met with the stoma care nurse.
Research by Chaudhri et al (2005) shows that the long term effect of stoma education is more effective if provided in the preoperative setting. It enables patients to attain proficiency in managing their stomas sooner and reduces postoperative stay.
Haugen et al (2006) have shown a direct correlation between the experiencing of the preoperative counselling and the long term adjustment to life with the stoma. The better the counselling, the easier the adjustment.
The review by Brown and Randle (2005) looked into the impact of stoma surgery on the patient's life and the implications thereof for nursing in practice. It shows that nurses play a key role, both pre- and postoperative. Baxter and Salter state that stoma care nurses offer support concerning processing and accepting the diagnosis and prognosis, adjustment to life with a

stoma, acquiring practical skills and dealing with issues with regard to family and friends, body image and sexuality (Baxter and Salter in Brown and Randle, 2005).

Colwell and Gray (2007) also conclude that preoperative preparation by a stoma care nurse has a positive influence on the postoperative results: quality of life, skills and long term adjustment to life with a stoma.

Wu et al (2007) examined the relationship between self-efficacy and quality of life, and the results indicated that these variables were positively correlated. Self-efficacy is an important factor to consider in the provision of care to the stoma patient. Stoma care nurses can, by motivating patients to manage their stoma through offering support and providing information, enhance self-care and self-confidence in patients.

Research by Fiorovanti (1988) also showed that proper information has a positive influence on the adjustment in the period after surgery. Patients who are better informed have less trouble in adjusting emotionally, socially, sexually, as well as in behaviour and stoma management.

Recommendation 13: (as concluded from the abovementioned)
Provide stoma information and counselling in the preoperative phase.

Conclusion Level 2	
level	**Author title**
B	Millan, M. (2009) Preoperative stoma siting and education by stomatherapists of colorectal cancer patients: a descriptive study in twelve Spanish colorectal units. *Colorectal disease, 12,* 88-92.
B	Chaudhri, S., Brown, L., Hassan, H. & Horgan, A.F. (2005). Preoperative intensive, community-based vs. traditional stoma education: a randomized, controlled trial. *Diseases of the Colon & Rectum, 48(3),* 504-509.
B	Haugen, V., Bliss, D.Z. & Savik, K. (2006). Perioperative factors that affect long-term adjustment to an incontinent ostomy. *Journal of Wound Ostomy Continence Nursing, 33 (5),* 525-535.
B	Brown, H. & Randle, J. (2005). Living with a stoma: a review of the literature. *Journal of clinical nursing, 14,* 74-81.
C	Colwell, J.C. & Gray, M. (2007). Does preoperative teaching and stoma site marking affect surgical outcomes in patients undergoing ostomy surgery? *Journal of wound ostomy continence nursing, 34(5),* 492-496.
C	Fioravanti, M., Di Cesare, F., Ramelli, L., La Torre, F., Nicastro, A., Messinetti, S. & Lazzari, R. (1988). Pre-surgery information and psychological adjustment to enterostomy. *The Italian Journal of Surgical Science, 18(1),* 55- 61.
C	Wu, H.K.M., Chau, J.P.C. & Twinn, S., (2007). Self-efficacy and quality of life among stoma patients in Hong Kong. *Cancer Nursing, 30(3),* 186-193.

4.2.A.1. Preoperative consultation

During the preoperative consultation, a number of issues will be identified and explained. The sequence and extent may vary per consultation and will be determined by the stoma care nurse together with the patient and spouse or relatives. The stoma care nurse explains her function, the purpose of the consultation and the duration. The nurse checks with the patient if the personal information in his file is correct. The stoma care nurse then verifies what information the patient received, regarding his illness and treatment, from his attending physician. The patient's expectations are also discussed.

The nurse is able to adapt the information to the needs, wishes and cognitive skills of the patient.

The research report "Quality and organization of the ostomy" (NSV, 2009 c) looked into the degree of satisfaction patients experienced with regard to the provision of information on various topics. Varying per topic, between twenty to thirty percent of respondents indicated having received insufficient information. This advocates use of a checklist during the consultation, to ensure that all topics are addressed.

During consultation general stoma information, substantiated explanations related to the planned operation, the consequences of having a stoma, stoma management and information about appliances are discussed. Appendix VI specifies all the subjects that should be discussed.

Recommendation 14: (as concluded from the abovementioned)
Provide the patient with information during the preoperative consultation with regard to receiving a stoma and the consequences for everyday life.

Conclusion Level 3	
level	Author title
C	Nederlandse Stomavereniging (2009c). *Kwaliteit en organisatie van stomazorg. Onderzoeksverslag in opdracht van de NSV* . Amsterdam: Newcom Research & Consultancy B.V. Kapteijns, A. & Buitinga, S.

4.2.A.2. Spouse and relatives

When providing preoperative counselling it is advised to involve a spouse or relative.

Persson et al (2005 a) indicate that providing counselling is as important to relatives as it is to the patient. Relatives need to be treated with respect and should be involved in the daily routines. She concludes that there is need for information and participation on the part of the patient's relatives and that there is still a discrepancy between what is being offered and what is needed or understood. To further optimize the quality of care, more attention should be paid to the various aspects of information and participation in the care for both the patient and the relatives. By encouraging relatives to be more involved incomprehension or dissatisfaction at a later stage can be prevented.

Cotrim and Pereira (2008) have investigated the impact of colorectal cancer on patients (with and without a stoma) and their relatives. One of the outcomes was that carers of stoma patients are more depressed and anxious compared to carers of patients without stoma. This anxiety is being projected back to the patient.

Northouse et al (1999) examined how patients and their spouses can be supported in coming to terms with the diagnosis, the treatment and the consequences thereof. Conclusion of this study is that spouses should be involved in counselling and education because they tend to be more negative towards the situation than the patient is. Both especially require information on the expected course of recovery, coaching in making the necessary adjustments and need to learn coping with the effects of the treatment.

Conclusion Level 3	
level	Author title
B	Cotrim, H. & Pereira, G. (2008). Impact of colorectal cancer on patient and family: implications for care. *European journal of oncology nursing, 12,* 217- 226.
C	Persson, E. , Gustavsson, B., Hellström, A.L., Fridstedt, G., Lappas, G. & Hultén, L. (2005a). Information to the relatives of people with ostomies. *Journal of Wound Ostomy Continence Nursing, 32 (4),* 238-245.
+	Northouse, L.L., Schafer, J.A., Tipton, J. & Metivier, L. (1999). The concerns of patients and spouses after the diagnosis of colon cancer: a qualitative analysis. *Journal of Wound Ostomy Continence Nursing, 26 (1),* 8-17.

Recommendation 15: (as concluded from the abovementioned)
The spouse and/or relatives of the stoma patient should be involved in preoperative education.

4.2.B. Stoma site marking
The second element of the preoperative preparation concerns appointing and marking the stoma site.
Finding the best place for a stoma contributes to the best possible quality of life after surgery; it prevents problems and saves costs.
The stoma site should always be marked preoperatively by the stoma care nurse. Always means: prior to operations where it is certain that a stoma will be constructed, as well as prior to operations where a stoma may possibly be constructed.
Literature shows that most problems in stomata are caused by incorrect siting. According to Brand and Dujovny (2008), this can be prevented by proper preoperative planning, involving the surgeon, the stoma care nurse as well as the patient.
A retrospective comparative study by Bass et al (1997) shows that patients suffer more complications when preoperative stoma siting was not performed. This also includes early complications that result in longer hospitalisation. It is plausible that more complications also lead to higher costs (Bass et al, 1997).
These findings are consistent with those of Turnbull (2002). The preoperative procedure of marking the stoma site positively influences the clinical and financial outcomes for patients with a stoma. A poorly placed stoma can result in failure of the pouching system, skin and leakage problems, and may require either local revision or relocation of the stoma. These complications can also lead to an increase in the consumption of stoma appliances and accessories, higher costs associated with patient care and negatively impact the quality of the patient's life (Millan, 2009; Brand and Dujovny, 2008; Cataldo, 2008).
Stoma construction and care not only require excellent surgical techniques, but preoperative care also implies the marking of an appropriate stoma site. Patients who are scheduled for surgery, with the prospect of a possible stoma construction, are referred to the stoma care nurse. The stoma care nurse will determine the best site. Locations should be chosen carefully and be marked as a guideline for the surgeon (Rozen, 1997).
According to Berry in the ACRS Document (2007), stoma siting should preferably be done by stoma care nurses or surgeons skilled in colorectal surgery.
The final location is determined by the surgeon during the operation in which the condition of the bowel is a co- factor.

Situations can occur where the stoma care nurse will take initiative to determine a stoma site, based on specific knowledge and responsibility and without the request of a specialist. However, the stoma care nurse will always inform the specialist.

Recommendation 16: (as concluded from the abovementioned)
Ensure that preoperative siting of the stoma becomes a standard procedure, which is always done in consultation with the patient. This has to be done with every patient who has to undergo surgery where a stoma will definitely or possibly be constructed.

Conclusion Level 2	
level	Author title
B	Millan, M. (2009) Preoperative stoma siting and education by stomatherapists of colorectal cancer patients: a descriptive study in twelve Spanish colorectal units. *Colorectal disease, 12,* 88-92.
B	Bass, E.M., Del Pino, A., Tan, A., Pearl, R.K., Orsay, C.P. & Abcarian, H. (1997). Does preoperative stoma marking and education by the enterostomal therapist affect outcome? *Diseases of the Colon & Rectum, 40(4),* 440-442.
D	Brand, M.I. & Dujovny, N. (2008). Preoperative considerations and creation of normal ostomies. *Clinics in colon and rectal surgery, 21(1),* 5-16.
D	Turnbull, G.B. (2002). The stoma care files: the position on preoperative stoma site positioning. *Vancouver stoma care high life, 41(1)* , 1,14.
D	Cataldo, P.A. (2008) Technical tips for stoma creation in the challenging patient. *Clinics in colon and rectal surgery, 21(1),* 17-22.
D	Rozen, B.L. (1997).The value of a well-placed stoma. *Cancer practice, 5(6),* 347-352.
D	ASCRS and WOCN Society (2007). Joint position statement on the value of preoperative stoma. Marking for patients undergoing faecal ostomy surgery. *Journal of Wound, Ostomy and Continence Nursing, 34(6),* 627-8.

4.2.B.1. Method

Brand and Dujovny (2008) state that most problems in stoma management are caused by poor siting. This can be prevented by proper preoperative planning by the specialist, stoma care nurse as well as the patient. They, as well as Bass et al (1997) state that the position of the stoma should be chosen in such a way that the patient is able to manage his stoma independently and resume normal life after recovery. The ideal site meets the following requirements: the stoma is visible to the patient; appliances can be safely applied and also provides optimal freedom of movement.
In the study by Bass et al (1997) the site is determined in three positions: supine, sitting and standing, then locating a stable flat area on the abdomen the size of a skin barrier, visible and accessible to the patient.
The stoma should be placed at the superior apex of the infra-umbilical fat fold in the lower quadrant to improve the visibility of the stoma to the patient (Turnbull, 2002, Brand and Dujovny, 2008). The stoma opening should pass through the rectus abdominus to reduce the likelihood of a parastomal hernia or stomal prolaps (Brand and Dujovny, 2008). The American Society of Colon and Rectal Surgeons (ASCRS) and the Wound Ostomy Continence Care Nurses Society (WOCN) together developed a procedure for locating the stoma site (2007). They describe a

number of key points that correspond to aspects from previously mentioned literature, amongst others Rozen (1997), Millan (2009), Brand and Dujovny (2008) and Cataldo (2008). These aspects are:

Positional aspects such as contractures, build and mobility (wheelchair dependent).

Physical considerations are large protruding or hanging abdomen, abdominal folds, wrinkles, scars, other stomata, straight abdominal muscle, waist, hip bone, sagging breasts, vision, mobility and herniation.

Patient related considerations mentioned are: diagnosis, clothing aspects, corset, radiotherapy history, age and activities.

Even the preferences of the medical specialist, preferences of the patient, type of stoma and the expected stool consistency are of influence.

If more than one stoma is necessary, the marking for colo- and urostomata should be placed at different horizontal planes/lines.

The method has been summarised in Appendix VII.

Recommendation 17: (as concluded from the abovementioned)
When locating the stoma site, take into account positional issues, physical and patient-related considerations and preferences of the patient and medical specialist.

Conclusion Level 2	
level	Author title
B	Millan, M. (2009) Preoperative stoma siting and education by stomatherapists of colorectal cancer patients: a descriptive study in twelve Spanish colorectal units. *Colorectal disease, 12,* 88-92.
B	Bass, E.M., Del Pino, A., Tan, A., Pearl, R.K., Orsay, C.P. & Abcarian, H. (1997). Does preoperative stoma marking and education by the enterostomal therapist affect outcome? *Diseases of the Colon & Rectum, 40(4),* 440-442.
D	Brand, M.I. & Dujovny, N. (2008). Preoperative considerations and creation of normal ostomies. *Clinics in colon and rectal surgery, 21(1),* 5-16.
D	Turnbull, G.B. (2002). The stoma care files: the position on preoperative stoma site positioning. *Vancouver stoma care high life, 41(1),* 1, 14.
D	Cataldo, P.A. (2008) Technical tips for stoma creation in the challenging patient. *Clinics in colon and rectal surgery, 21(1),* 17-22.
D	Rozen, B.L. (1997).The value of a well-placed stoma. *Cancer practice, 5(6),* 347-352.
D	ASCRS and WOCN Society (2007). Joint position statement on the value of preoperative stoma. Marking for patients undergoing fecal stoma care surgery. *Journal of Wound, Ostomy and Continence Nursing, 34(6),* 627-8.

4.2.B.2. Method in obese patients

Additional attention should be paid to determining the stoma site in an obese patient: Brand and Dujovny (2008) advise to mark the stoma site above the umbilicus. The stoma is more visible and easier to manage, which is not possible if the standard method is applied. Moreover, the hypodermic fat layer is less thick above the umbilicus than below the umbilicus (Cataldo, 2008).

Recommendation 18: (as concluded from the abovementioned)
In the case of an obese stomach, mark the stoma site, in consultation with the patient, above the umbilicus.

Conclusion Level 4	
level	Author title
D	Brand, M.I. & Dujovny, N. (2008). Preoperative considerations and creation of normal ostomies. *Clinics in colon and rectal surgery, 21(1),* 5-16.
D	Cataldo, P.A. (2008) Technical tips for stoma creation in the challenging patient. *Clinics in colon and rectal surgery, 21(1),* 17-22.

4.2.C. Opportunity to wear and practice with stoma appliances

The third element of the preoperative preparation concerns stoma appliances and the opportunity to see it and practice with it.

According to the report "Kwaliteit en organisatie van stomazorg" (NSV, 2009 c), nearly three-quarters of the respondents who had the opportunity to practice with stoma appliances, regarded it as a positive experience.

The previously mentioned study of Chaudri et al (2005), which showed that information in the preoperative phase is more effective, there was also opportunity in the preoperative phase for practising. It should however be kept in mind that the study of Chaudri et al was focused on the preoperative education in the home situation.

Pieper and Mikols (1996) did research on issues which worries or concerns the stoma patient. It is indicated that, although this is not always possible, preference goes out to start practicing in the preoperative phase.

Readding (2005) recommends encouraging patients to see, feel or wear, and be informed on, the different types of stoma bags that best fits the situation of the patient.

Recommendation 19: (as concluded from the abovementioned)
Discuss with the patient whether he wants to see, apply and/or remove different stoma appliances in the preoperative phase.

Conclusion Level 3	
level	Author title
B	Chaudhri, S., Brown, L., Hassan, H. & Horgan, A.F. (2005). Preoperative intensive, community-based vs. traditional stoma education: a randomized, controlled trial. *Diseases of the Colon & Rectum, 48(3),* 504-509.
C	Pieper, B. & Mikols, C. (1996). Predischarge and postdischarge concerns of persons with an ostomy. *Journal of wound ostomy continence nursing, 23(2),* 105-109.
C	Nederlandse Stomavereniging (2009c). *Kwaliteit en organisatie van stomazorg. Onderzoeksverslag in opdracht van de NSV* . Amsterdam: Newcom Research & Consultancy B.V. Kapteijns, A. & Buitinga, S.
D	Readding, L.A. (2005). Hospital to home, smoothing the journey for the new ostomist. *British journal of nursing, 14(16),* 16-20.

	Recommendation	Conclusion level
13	Provide stoma information and counselling the preoperative phase.	2
14	Provide the patient with information during the preoperative consultation with regard to receiving a stoma and the consequences for everyday life.	3
15	The spouse and/or relatives of the stoma patient should be involved in preoperative education.	3
16	Ensure that preoperative siting of the stoma becomes a standard procedure, which is always done in consultation with the patient. This has to be done with every patient who has to undergo surgery where a stoma will definitely or possibly be constructed.	2
17	When locating the stoma site, take into account positional issues, physical and patient-related considerations and preferences of the patient and medical specialist.	2
18	In the case of an obese stomach, mark the stoma site, in consultation with the patient, above the umbilicus.	4
19	Discuss with the patient whether he wants to see, apply and/or remove different stoma appliances in the preoperative phase.	3

Chapter 5 Postoperative phase and discharge phase

The postoperative phase is described in this chapter. The questions taken from the analysis of the problem areas that will be answered in this chapter are:
- "What is understood by standard stoma care in the postoperative phase and discharge phase?",
- " Complications of stoma construction in the postoperative phase and discharge phase: definitions, prevention, recognition, identification and treatment".
- "Choice of appliances in the postoperative phase: when to use which appliance?"
After having defined this phase, three more subjects will be addressed: what does standard stoma care in this phase comprise of, the complications of this phase the use of appliances.

5.1. Definitions
The working group determined the following definitions of these phases:
Postoperative phase: the phase from the operation until discharge from hospital.
Discharge Phase: phase in which discharge from hospital is prepared.
These phases overlap and together form the clinical phase.
Definitions relating to appliances:
Stoma appliances: skin barrier and stoma bag.
Skin Barrier: the adhesive part of the stoma appliance.
Stoma bag: the part of the stoma appliance that collects the output.
Stoma accessories: all devices (except stoma appliances) that may be required for stoma management.

5.2. Standard stoma care in the postoperative clinical phase
In regard to stoma care in the postoperative phase, a number of elements can be distinguished:
A. Observations.
B. Guidance to self-care.
C. Intervention in different situations or complications.

5.2.A. Observations
The following is a general description of the points of attention in the postoperative phase. Appendix VIII provides a point by point description of what is considered to be normal in this phase.
After surgery, the stoma needs to be controlled and assessed on a number of points, starting immediately after surgery. During the first 24-48 hours after surgery, these points should be assessed at least every eight hours, thereafter the observation frequency decreases.
Several authors identify the topics: Vujnovich (2008) mentions colour, output, bridge in place, skin condition, size of the stoma, sutures, and temperature. Erwin-Toth (2006) mentions examination of the stoma, vitality of stomal mucosa and surrounding skin, sutures and surgery wound. Burch (2005 b) describes oedema and, correspondingly, the size of the stoma, stoma colour, temperature of the stoma, sutures, output and normal postoperative output pattern.
The working group summarised the main observations in the first days after surgery as follows:

vitality of the stoma on the basis of colour, aspect of the mucous membrane and oedema, height and size, location, whether or not a bridge in place, sutures, splints (urostomy), stoma appliances, condition of the peristomal skin, functioning of intestines or kidneys on the basis of production and flatus.

If the splints (urostomy) do not produce, consult with the urologist. The urologist could advise to rinse.

See Appendix VIII for all postoperative observations.

Recommendation 20: (as concluded from the abovementioned)
Perform specific observations relating to the stoma immediately after surgery until the first 48 hours. These observations should be performed at least every eight hours.

Conclusion Level 4	
level	**Author title**
D	Vujnovich, A. (2008) Pre and post- operative assessment of patients with a stoma. *Nursing standard, 22(19),* 50-56.
D	Erwin-Toth, P. (2006). Ostomy care and rehabilitation in colorectal cancer. *Seminars in oncology nursing, 22(3),* 174-177.
D	Burch, J. (2005b). The pre- and postoperative nursing care for patients with a stoma. *British Journal of Nursing, 14(6),* 310-318.

To be able to observe the stoma properly, Fullham (2008), Burch (2005 b) and Erwin-Toth (2006) advise to use transparent stoma appliances in this phase.

Recommendation 21: (as concluded from the abovementioned)
Make sure that transparent stoma material is applied so that postoperative stoma observations can be performed properly.

Conclusion Level 4	
level	**Author title**
D	Fulham, J. (2008a). A guide to caring for patients with a newly formed stoma in the acute hospital setting. *Gastrointestinal Nursing, 6(8),* 14-23.
D	Erwin-Toth, P., (2006). Ostomy care and rehabilitation in colorectal cancer. *Seminars in oncology nursing, 22(3),* 174-177.
D	Burch, J. (2005 b). The pre- and postoperative nursing care for patients with a stoma. *British journal of nursing, 14(6),* 310-318.

5.2.B. Guidance towards self-care

After surgery, it is decided together with the patient when he would be able to start to learn stoma management. The starting point for teaching self-care is that the patient is able to take care of his stoma by himself. The time it takes to achieve this, is dependent on the individual. The stoma care nurse has to take into account the physical and psychological situation at the time. Erwin-Toth (2006) believes that the patient must be willing to learn. If the patient is unwilling or claims to be unable to learn self-care, the stoma care nurse will have to motivate him with good reasons on the importance of learning self-care and to start with this as soon as possible after surgery (Erwin-Toth, 2006). The stoma management should be integrated in the daily routine during the clinical phase. In this regard the ward nurses play an important role. The use of illustrations can be supportive in the teaching-learning of the self-care process.

Black (2004) notes that the best time to discuss the anxieties and concerns of the patient regarding the acceptance of the stoma, by himself as well as his environment, is during teaching and learning stoma care. A private space (one-on-one-situation) is very important. Learning self-care is essential for the processing and acceptance of the stoma.

A digital or paper roadmap is used in teaching self-care. The patient's progress in the learning process can be recorded in this plan, as well as the stage of self-care that has been reached. The reason why a particular step has not been achieved, can also been noted (see Appendix IX).

O'Connor (2005) states that a patient should only be discharged from hospital if he has sufficient stoma management skills. Regardless whether the stoma is temporary or permanent, every patient needs a basic level of skills and knowledge.

Recommendation 22: (as concluded from the abovementioned)
Provide active support or co-ordinate self-care teaching. Adapt the pace of teaching self-care to each individual stoma patient.

Conclusion Level 4	
level	**Author title**
D	Black, P.K. (2004). Psychological, sexual and cultural issues for patients with a stoma. *British journal of nursing, 13(12),* 692-697.
D	O'Connor, G. (2005). Teaching stoma-management skills: the importance of selfcare. *British journal of nursing, 14(4),* 320-324
D	Erwin-Toth, P. (2006). Ostomy care and rehabilitation in colorectal cancer. *Seminars in oncology nursing, 22(3),* 174-177.

5.2.B.1. Spouse and relatives

Also in this phase, the spouse and/or relatives are involved, since this is in the best interest of the patient. Persson et al (2005a) describe that both the patient and his relatives acknowledge the importance of various aspects of information and care to the family. Erwin-Toth (2006) on the other hand, warns that this involvement should not create a situation in which the patient becomes dependent on others for managing his stoma.

Stuchfield describes (in O 'Connor, 2005) that patients find it reassuring when family or relatives also receive instruction on stoma care, so they can support the patient if he needs help, especially in the first period after discharge from hospital.

Northouse et al (1999) also state that spouses indicate an increased involvement in care than before the patient became ill.

Recommendation 23: (as concluded from the abovementioned)
In consultation with the stoma patient, the spouse and/or relatives should be involved in the process of learning to take care of the stoma.

Conclusion Level 3	
level	Author title
C	Persson, E., Gustavsson, B., Hellström, A.L., Fridstedt, G., Lappas, G. & Hultén, L. (2005a). Information to the relatives of people with ostomies. *Journal of Wound Ostomy Continence Nursing, 32(4)*, 238-245.
D	O'Connor,G. (2005). Teaching stoma-management skills: the importance of selfcare. *British journal of nursing, 14(4)*, 320-324
D	Erwin-Toth, P., (2006). Ostomy care and rehabilitation in colorectal cancer. *Seminars in oncology nursing, 22(3)*, 174-177.
+	Northouse, L.L., Schafer, J.A., Tipton, J. & Metivier, L. (1999). The concerns of patients and spouses after the diagnosis of colon cancer: a qualitative analysis. *Journal of Wound Ostomy Continence Nursing, 26(1)*, 8-17.

5.2.B.2. Discharge Phase

As described, the discharge phase is part of the clinical phase. During the discharge phase preparations, with regard to the transition of stoma care from hospital to the home situation, are made.

The stoma care nurse determines to what extent the patient is able to take care of his stoma. This is done by asking the patient to demonstrate his competency in practical skills. (Steinaker and Bell in O'Connor, 2005). At the same time it enables the stoma care nurse to check the stoma and the peristomal skin. Together with the patient and relatives, she then determines what care is required after discharge from hospital. Starting point is independent stoma management by the patient. If this goal was not achieved during the clinical phase, it is to be continued within the home situation. It is advisable to turn to community care, with knowledge of stoma care, for support in the home situation.

A written transfer is issued for community care, care providers or nursing personnel of the institution where the patient might (temporary) stay. O'Connor (2005) indicates that an organized exchange of information between hospital and community will ensure that education and support are continued following discharge from hospital. (See Appendix XIV for the contents of transferring.)

The stoma care nurse ensures that the required stoma care appliances are ordered. She explains to relatives how to order and which appliances are reimbursed. If necessary, appliances for the first day(s) can be issued. From a study by Haugen et al (2006) it became apparent that concerns about acquiring stoma appliances is of one of the factors that negatively influences the long-term adaptation to a stoma. Taylor (1999 in Readding, 2005) too states that patient satisfaction with the appliances is important and promotes rehabilitation.

Shortly before leaving the hospital, there will be a discharge consultation. All relevant information will once again be discussed briefly and patient and relatives' understanding of all issues is double-checked. Readding (2005) describes that it is important to clearly explain to the patient what is implied by "normal", referring to the observations of the stoma (see Appendix XV). Potter (2000) indicates that it is important for the patient to be well-informed about the normal functioning of his particular stoma.

Patients with an ileostomy should be given information on the possibility of medication not being optimally absorbed due to the accelerated passage or the shortened length of the functional bowel.

At discharge, a follow-up appointment with the stoma care nurse is made and the accessibility of the stoma care nurse is explained and a contact phone number given in writing.

The stoma care nurse explains and justifies why postoperative check-ups are crucial. Research by Herlufsen et al (2006) showed that 38 percent of patients with a skin disorder do not recognize it as such. Also, 80 percent of patients with a skin disorder did not seek help from a professional. Readding (2005) states that telephone consultation can be useful for uncomplicated questions, but also to help identify more complex problems.

Appendix XI has a checklist with the points of attention for discharge, which can be used by the stoma care nurse in this phase.

Recommendation 24: (as concluded from the abovementioned)
In the discharge phase, in consultation with the stoma patient, all aspects that need to be taken care of before being discharged from hospital, should be checked systematically.

Conclusion Level 3	
level	Author title
B	Haugen, V., Bliss, D.Z. & Savik, K. (2006). Perioperative factors that affect long-term adjustment to an incontinent ostomy. *Journal of Wound Ostomy Continence Nursing, 33(5)*, 525-535.
C	Herlufsen, P., Olsen, A.G., Carlsen, B., Nybaek, H., Karlsmark, T., Laursen, T.N. & Jemec, G.B.E. (2006). OstomySkin study: a study of peristomal skin disorders in patients with permanent stomas. *British Journal of Nursing, 15(16)*, 854-862.
D	O'Connor, G. (2005). Teaching stoma-management skills: the importance of selfcare. *British journal of nursing, 14(4)*, 320-324
D	Readding, L.A. (2005). Hospital to home, smoothing the journey for the new ostomist. *British journal of nursing, 14(16)*, 16-20.
D	Potter, K.L. (2000). Surgical oncology of the pelvis: ostomy planning and management. *Journal of Surgical oncology, 73*, 237-242.

5.2.C. Intervention in abnormal situations or during complications

The stoma care nurse has the task to recognize abnormalities from the normal situation or identify complications in this phase. Depending on the problem, the stoma care nurse will personally intervene, instruct the ward nurse or consult a medical specialist.

On the basis of her correct (theoretical) knowledge and experience, the stoma care nurse can determine whether intervention or consultation is necessary. The most common complications during the first phase after surgery and the actions to be carried out, are discussed further on in this chapter.

Besides the knowledge and skills of the stoma care nurse, there is another reason for regular contact with the patient during the clinical phase. Pringle and Swan (2001) describe that regular contact between the stoma care nurse and the patient and his family promotes restoring confidence, self-esteem and independence.

Recommendation 25: (as concluded from the abovementioned)
Ensure that the stoma care nurse is in charge of the stoma care in the postoperative phase.

Conclusion Level 3	
level	**Author title**
C	Pringle, W. & Swan, E. (2001). Continuing care after discharge from hospital for stoma patients. *British journal of nursing, 10(19),* 1275-1288

5.2.D. Food and fluid intake

Many ostomates and relatives have questions about food in connection with the stoma. Summarised it can be said that a person with an intestinal stoma does not need a special diet and is advised to follow a healthy, balanced and varied diet. People should be encouraged to enjoy their food, eat regularly and chew food carefully and/or cut it into small pieces (Fulham, 2008; Williams, 2007; Burch, 2006).

However, adjustments might be necessary. Certain food may have an effect on the production of stools, gas and odour.

In an ileostomy the intake of fluid and salt must be increased, compared to normal intake, because the reabsorption of moisture and salt (about six to eight grams of salt per litre of stool) in the colon is lost. It is therefore recommended that an ileostomate always has a consultation with a dietician. For better absorption of nutrients and moisture, Welink (2007) recommends to spread the intake of food and fluids (two to two and a half litres) over the entire day. When sleep is disturbed by stoma production, it may be advised to reduce the evening meal or to take a hot meal earlier in the day. (See Appendix XII for specific nutritional aspects and Appendix XIII for nutrition-related complications.)

Recommendation 26: (as concluded from the abovementioned)
Provide the stoma patient with general recommendations on healthy eating.

Recommendation 27: (as concluded from the abovementioned)
Ensure that the ileostomy patient, prior to discharge from the hospital, is given information by a dietician on fluid intake, nutrition and consumption of extra salt.

Conclusion Level 4	
level	**Author title**
D	Williams, J. (2007). Stoma care nursing: what the community nurse needs to know. *British journal of community nursing, 12(8),* 342- 346
D	Fulham, J. (2008b).Providing dietary advice for the individual with a stoma. *British Journal of Nursing, 17(2),* 22-27.
D	Burch, J. (2006). Nutrition and the ostomate: input, output and absorption. *British journal of community nursing, 11(8),* 349-351.
D	Welink- Lamberts B., Werkgroep CHIODAZ (2007). Nieuwe dieetbehandelings-richtlijn ileostomy. *Ned. Tijdschrift voor Voeding & Diëtiek 62(3),* 7-10

Fluid intake in urostomy

The European guideline "Incontinent urostomy" (EAUN, 2009) advises urostomates to ensure adequate fluid intake. In practice, this can be judged on the basis of the colour of the urine; it should be pale yellow or straw coloured.

Both Doughty (2005) and Fulham (2008) describe that adequate fluid intake is essential for prevention of urinary tract infection and strong urine odour. Doughty also advises to spread the fluid intake over the day.

Burch (2005a) describes that alkaline urine can cause crystal forming on or near the stoma. A slightly acidic pH of the urine can ensure that crystals will not be formed, and to achieve this cranberry can be used.

Tsukada et al (1994) conducted a study in a small group of urostomy patients on the influence of using cranberry. It was concluded that the acidity of the urine in the stoma bag was higher when cranberries were used. This group of people also suffered less skin disorders and the skin barrier was less affected.

Burch (2005a) also mentions that consumption of cranberry could reduce mucus forming from the urostomy.

The European Guideline on Incontinent Urostomy (2009) states that cranberry may have a positive effect on symptoms of urinary tract infection, odour, skin disorders or leakage.

Recommendation 28: (as concluded from the abovementioned)
Ensure that the urostomy patient receives adequate advice on required fluid intake, to achieve pale yellow or straw coloured urine.

Recommendation 29: (as concluded from the abovementioned)
Advise the urostomy patient about the remedial benefits of cranberry juice or capsules in the event of skin- or leakage problems or (symptomatic) urinary tract infections.

Conclusion Level 3	
level	**Author title**
C	Tsukada, K., Tokunaga, K., Iwama, T., Mishima, Y., Tazawa, K. & Fujimaki, M. (1994) Cranberry juice and its impact on peri-stomal skin conditions for urostomy patients. Os*tomy Wound Management, 40(9),* 60-68.
AGREE	European Association of Urology Nurses (2009). *Good practice in health care: incontinent urstomy.* European Association of Urology Nurses Geng, V., Cobussen, H., Fillingham, S., Holroyd, S., Kiesbye, B. & Vahr, S.
D	Burch, J. (2005a). Stoma complications encountered in the community, AZ. *British Journal of Community Nursing, 10(7),* 324-329.
D	Doughty, D. (2005). Principles of ostomy management in oncology patients. *The journal of supportive oncology, 3(1),* 59-69.

5.3. Complications in the postoperative clinical phase

The most common complications are being described in this section. The complications are divided into two groups: stoma problems and skin disorders.

Often a distinction is made between early and late complications; however, in the literature researched this distinction is not clear. Therefore it has been decided to describe the definitions of all the most common, relevant complications in this chapter. The rest of the information for each complication is described in Appendix XIII in terms of definition, characteristics, incidence, cause/risk factors, consequences, intervention by the nurse, treatment and prevention.

Cottam et al (2007) did research on the problems and complications in the first three weeks after surgery. They define a problematic stoma as a stoma which needs one or more accessories to keep the patient clean and dry for a minimum of 24 hours. She concludes in her study that the height of the stoma (<10 mm), type of stoma (ileostomy) and gender of the patient (female) are significant risk factors for the development of stoma problems. Also in emergency surgery, the risk of a problematic stoma is larger.

Cottam et al describe the most common problems in this period as retraction, separation, necrosis and prolapse. In three diagnoses where a stoma construction is needed (colorectal cancer, ulcerative colitis and a group of various reasons), a statistically significant impact on stoma problems were recorded (Cottam et al, 2007).

Colwell and Beitz (2007) did research to record data on stoma complications. The aim was to validate definitions and interventions in order to assess the incidence of complications. Until now, much has been published on these complications, but often in the form of case studies; there is no real evidence on the various complications. In this study, Colwell and Beitz validated the definitions as well as the interventions. In 5.3.1. the validated definitions are described and the remaining information per complication can be found in Appendix XIII.

Recommendation 30: (as concluded from the abovementioned)
Use clear, validated descriptions of the complications. Work from these valid definitions to further uniformity in nursing interventions.

Conclusion Level 3	
level	Author title
C	Colwell, J.C. & Beitz, J. (2007). Survey of wound, ostomy and continence (WOC) nurse clinicians on stomal and peristomal complications: a content validation study. *Journal of Wound Ostomy Continence Nursing, 34(1),* 57-69.
C	Cottam, J., Richards, A., Hasted, A. & Blackman, A. (2006). Results of a nationwide prospective audit of stoma complications within 3 weeks of surgery. *Colorectal Disease, 9(9),* 834-838

5.3.1. Stomal complications

The most common and relevant stomal complications are defined and described in this paragraph, as validated by Colwell and Beitz (2007).

Complication	Definition
Parastomal (peristomal) hernia	A defect in abdominal fascia that allows the intestine to bulge into the parastomal area.
Stoma prolapse	Telescoping of the intestine through the stoma.
Stoma necrosis	Death of the stomal tissue resulting from impaired blood flow.
Mucocutaneous separation	The detachment of stomal tissue from the surrounding peristomal skin.
Stoma retraction	The disappearance of normal stoma protrusion in line with or below skin level.
Stoma stenosis	Impairment of effluent drainage due to narrowing or contracting of the stoma tissue at skin or fascia level.
Stoma trauma	Injury to the stoma mucosa often related to pressure or physical force.
Stoma fistula	An abnormal communication between the stoma and surrounding tissue or skin.

5.3.2. Peristomal complications

The definitions of the most common and relevant skin disorders, as validated by Colwell and Beitz (2007) are described in this paragraph.

Complication	Definition
Peristomal irritant contact dermatitis	Damage resulting from skin exposure to faecal or urinary drainage or chemical preparation.
Peristomal suture granuloma	Excessive tissue occurring at skin/stoma base in areas of retained or reactive suture material.
Peristomal candidiasis:	An overgrowth of fungal organisms (Candida) sufficient to cause inflammation, infection or skin disease in the peristomal area.
Peristomal folliculitis	An inflammation of hair follicles on the peristomal skin caused by Staphylococcus aureus.
Pseudo verrucous lesions	Wart-like lesions in the peristomal area related to chronic moisture exposure and irritation.
Persistomal pyoderma gangrenosum	An ulcerative skin condition of unknown etiology occurring around a stoma.
Peristomal varices	Large portosystemic venous collateral blood vessels occurring at the site of the stoma

5.3.2.1. Measuring instruments

Measuring instruments have been developed in recent years to enable the description of skin disorders in a stoma. The purpose of these instruments is to classify and diagnose peristomal skin disorders and to describe these problems uniformly. All stoma care professionals will thus be able to describe skin disorders in the same manner. The measuring instruments that are currently being used in the Netherlands are the Ostomy Skin Tool (consisting DET score and the AIM guide) and the SACS ™ instrument. There are no comparative studies on these instruments and therefore not possible to recommend one of them over the other.

It is beyond the scope of this guideline to assess the different instruments in order to make a recommendation on what instrument should be used. However, the working group is of the opinion that the use of one particular measuring instrument on (inter)national level could improve the quality and reliability of classification of skin disorders. Such a step can be considered as a start to consistent intervention in such skin disorders.

Recommendation 31: (as concluded from the abovementioned)
Use a measuring instrument for describing and diagnosing peristomal skin disorders.

5.3.3. Other problems with the stoma

Problem	Definition
Leakage	Faeces or urine leaks out between the skin and the skin barrier as result of a complication or other problem.
Pancaking	Faeces does not move down into the stoma bag, but remains around the stoma.
Oedema	Accumulation of fluid in the stoma, causing the stoma to become bigger.
High output production in bowel stoma	Production exceeding 1 litre per 24 hours.
Obstipation	Accumulation of faeces in the colon, resulting in a delayed excretion of hard, dry stools through the stoma.
Obstruction	Blockage of the stoma passage leading to no stool and/or flatus.
Excessive gas forming	Gas forming to such an extent that the ostomate feels constrained.

Leakage is a common problem experienced by stoma patients and it is the task of the stoma care nurse to detect the cause of the leakage.

Herlufsen et al (2006) describe that stoma patients often don't recognize the symptoms of the leakage as a potential problem which only worsens the problem. If the leakage is experienced as a problem, the skin barrier is taped on the outer edge, which is a false solution that may actually exacerbate the problem. Because faecal matter or urine remains on the skin under the skin barrier longer, the skin becomes increasingly irritated (contact dermatitis) and the problem enters into a vicious circle.

Readding (2005), Rolstad and Erwin-Toth (2010) and Redmond et al (2009) advocate good counselling and teaching. Being able to recognize the symptoms of (potential) problems can be enhanced by providing the patient with solid information.

High output, obstipation, obstruction or excessive gas may be indicators of potential bowel movement pattern problems. A highly inconsistent pattern can also cause problems.

Recommendation 32: (as concluded from the abovementioned)
Ensure the stoma patient is aware of the symptoms related to the various potential complications or problems.

Conclusion Level 3	
level	**Author title**
C	Redmond, C., Cowin, C. & Parker, T. (2009). The experience of faecal leakage among ileostomists. *British Journal of Nursing, 18(17),* 12-17.
C	Herlufsen, P., Olsen, A.G., Carlsen, B., Nybaek, H., Karlsmark, T., Laursen, T.N. & Jemec, G.B.E. (2006). OsomySkin study: a study of peristomal skin disorders in patients with permanent stomas. *British Journal of Nursing, 15(16),* 854-862.
D	Readding, L.A. (2005). Hospital to home, smoothing the journey for the new ostomist. *British journal of nursing, 14(16),* 16-20.
D	Rolstad, B.S. & Erwin-Toth PL (2010). Peristomal skin complications: prevention and management. *American journal of nursing, 110 (2),* 43-48.

5.4. Choice of appliances: postoperative

Selecting and choosing appliances already starts in the preoperative phase. During preoperative counselling, the patient was informed about the difference between a one-piece and a two-piece appliance, given the opportunity to try them out and to state his preference for either the one-piece or the two-piece appliance. After surgery, an assessment is done whether the preference of the patient is feasible. According to Pontieri-Lewis (2006) the stoma appliance is intended to collect the stoma output and protect the skin. The stoma appliance should be odourless, comfortable, discreet and live up to the expected wear time, depending on the type of appliance (Pontieri-Lewis, 2006). Selection of the appliance is based on different criteria. Erwin-Toth (2006) describes stoma type, output, form of the abdomen and patient related factors such as vision, dexterity and personal preferences. Colwell and Beitz (2007) state that the wear time of the appliance (how often it must be changed) is determined by various factors such as the stoma and the area around the stoma (also see considerations in locating a site). Potter (2000) indicates that the stoma care nurse has the expertise to assist the patient in choosing the correct stoma appliance.

In the research on the use of stoma appliances by the Dutch Ostomy Association (NSV, 2010b) ostomates were asked about their expectations of stoma appliances. The three main aspects pointed out by the ostomates were security/safety, easy to use and odourless. There are differences between the different types of stomata and pouching systems (one-piece or two-piece).

In 2007, a working group of the V&VN Stoma care nurses designed a decision tree for choosing the appropriate appliances; see Appendix X. It contains the aspects which play a role in the choice of stoma appliances (skin barrier and stoma bag). This decision tree gives insight into the underlying reasons for the choice of appliance in each individual case. Summarised, the patient characteristics, personal preferences and stomal characteristics are examined. From this the product requirements are defined and a product can be selected. The skin barrier features to be selected from are: type of material, top layer, protective layer of the adhesive layer, model, size, opening and design: flat or convex. The features of the bag are: type of material, size, shape, colour, fasteners, filter, and method of attachment to the skin barrier. When choosing appliances the starting point should be that stoma care is made as uncomplicated as possible, which is in turn beneficial to mastering self-care.

In 2011 a new approach in the process of choosing a proper appliance was initiated in the Netherlands. The performance-oriented claim on stoma aids means that an assessment is done to decide which appliance is most suitable for the specific situation of a patient. Hereby the ICF classification was used. At the time of writing, this document was not yet complete.

Recommendation 33: (as concluded from the abovementioned)
Attempt to use a stoma appliance that best suits the characteristics of the stoma and the characteristics and personal preferences of the stoma patient.

Conclusion Level 3	
level	**Author title**
C	Colwell, J.C. & Beitz, J. (2007). Survey of wound, stoma care and continence (WOC) nurse clinicians on stomal and peristomal complications: a content validation study. *Journal of Wound Ostomy Continence Nursing, 34(1),* 57-69.
C	Nederlandse Stomavereniging (2010b). *Onderzoek naar het gebruik van stomamaterialen. Onderzoeksverslag in opdracht van de NSV.* Amsterdam: Newcom Research & Consultancy B.V. Kapteijns, A., Buitinga, S. & Meeusen, K.
D	Potter, K.L. (2000). Surgical oncology of the pelvis: ostomy planning and management. *Journal of Surgical oncology, 73,* 237-242.
D	Erwin-Toth, P. (2006). Ostomy care and rehabilitation in colorectal cancer. *Seminars in oncology nursing, 22(3),* 174-177
D	Pontieri-Lewis, V. (2006). Basics of ostomy care. *Medsurg nursing, 15(4),* 199-202.

5.4.1. Adjusting of the opening of the skin barrier

The stoma has a round or oval shape. Due to the increase and decrease of oedema after surgery the stoma will still change in size and shape. Therefore the opening of the skin barrier will have to be adjusted in this first period (two to three months after surgery). With each changing of the stoma appliance, changes to the size of the opening of the skin barrier must be monitored, and compared to previous checks (Pontieri-Lewis, 2006). Consequently, it may become necessary to select a different stoma appliance after a while. It is advisable to use a cut-to-fit skin barrier in this phase, and to use a stoma template, which can be adjusted when changes have to be made to the opening of the skin barrier.

Recommendation 34: (as concluded from the abovementioned)
Check regularly during three months after surgery, in consultation with the stoma patient, whether the opening of the skin barrier still fits the stoma. If necessary, adjust the stoma appliance.

Conclusion Level 4	
level	Author title
D	Pontieri-Lewis, V. (2006). Basics of ostomy care. *Medsurg nursing, 15(4)*, 199-202.

5.4.2. Flushable appliances and waste disposal

Ostomates have specific questions concerning the stoma appliances and accessories.
One of these questions concerns the disposal of waste. The used appliance can be placed in the normal household bin, preferably in a sealed disposable plastic bag. Additionally, ostomates can be informed on appliances that can be flushed down the toilet.
(Williams, 2007). These flushable stoma bags are only suitable for use by colostomates and since there is limited choice in flushable stoma bags, these may not be a practical alternative for all colostomates. However, they should be informed about this possibility.
McKenzie et al (2006) did research to discover if changing and disposing of (used) stoma appliances had any effect on the perceived psychological well-being of ostomates. Ostomates completed a questionnaire during the first four months after surgery. It was concluded that changing and disposing of stoma appliances affected the social activities of a small number of the ostomates. The author recommends that the stoma care nurse pays attention to this aspect.

Recommendation 35: (as concluded from the abovementioned)
Inform the stoma patient about the disposal of used stoma appliances.

Conclusion Level 4	
level	Author title
D	Williams, J. (2007). Stoma care nursing: what the community nurse needs to know. *British journal of community nursing, 12(8)*, 342- 346
D	McKenzie, F., White, C.A., Kendall, S., Finlayson, A., Urquhart, M. & Williams, I. (2006).Psychological impact of colostomy pouch change and disposal. *British Journal of Nursing, 15(6)*, 308 - 316.

5.4.3. Stoma accessories

Stoma accessories is the term used for all the aids that may be necessary in the care of the stoma, except for stoma appliances (skin barrier and stoma bag).
Rudoni and Dennis (2009) looked into the reasons for use of stoma accessories from both patients and stoma care nurses viewpoints. They also searched for evidence for the use of stoma accessories.
Reasons for using an aid are: painful skin, adhesion of the skin barrier, leakage, skin damage, hygiene and pain when removing the skin barrier, irregularities around the stoma, support of the abdominal wall, visibility of the stoma appliance, odour, pancaking and ballooning. Accessories

play an important role in improving the quality of life, both physically and psychologically. According to 72 percent of the participating stoma care nurses, assessment and advice by a stoma care nurse for implementing stoma accessories is considered necessary. On the other hand, 81,5 percent of participating ostomates are of the opinion that they can independently make decisions on stoma accessory use. This study showed that ostomates make use of stoma accessories based on their own insight more frequently when they are no longer in touch with their stoma care nurse. Research was also done into costs and whether these play a role in the use of stoma accessories. Ostomates indicated their awareness to the costs, but also that the use of accessories could be of importance to their psychological well-being. Nurses indicate that they consider the cost efficiency aspect, but do not hesitate to prescribe an aid when considered necessary to prevent skin disorders or for the ostomate's sense of self-confidence and protection. In the case of accessories too, use of them should be adapted to the individual situation of each ostomate (Rudoni and Dennis, 2009).

The working group is of the opinion that when choosing stoma accessories, the starting point should be making stoma management as simple as possible.

Recommendation 36: (as concluded from the abovementioned)
In the event of complications or problems, inform the stoma patient whether a stoma care aid is indicated and, if needed and in consultation with the stoma patient, make a choice from the accessories available.

Conclusion Level 4	
level	**Author title**
++	Rudoni, C. & Dennis, H. (2009) Accessories or necessities? Exploring consensus on usage of stoma accessories. *British journal of nursing, 18(18),* 1106-1112.

Many different stoma accessories are available in the Netherlands and these can be classified into the following groups:
Skin Protective solutions, fillers (stoma paste-products), products for the treatment of damaged skin (hydrocolloid powder), odour neutralizing agents, adhesives, glue solvents, fixatives, fixing means (belt or adhesive surface enlarging products), lubricant (anti-pancaking), mucus solvents (in urostomy), ventilation tools (filters/valve), other (such as push rings, fastening clips, flange). In addition, non-woven gauze and waste bags are used in stoma care. For adjusting the opening of the skin barrier a template and scissors or a punch can be used.
In the case of specific problems or complications (such as parastomal hernia or prolapse) an abdominal wall supporting accessory may be necessary; see the description of the complications. Also see Appendix XVI for generic descriptions of the different groups of stoma appliances and stoma accessories.

	Recommendation	Conclusion Level
20	Perform specific observations relating to the stoma immediately after surgery until the first 48 hours. These observations should be performed at least every eight hours.	4
21	Make sure that transparent stoma material is applied so that postoperative stoma observations can be performed properly.	4
22	Provide active support or co-ordinate self-care teaching. Adapt the pace of teaching self-care to each individual stoma patient.	4
23	In consultation with the stoma patient, the spouse and/or relatives should be involved in the process of learning to take care of the stoma.	3
24	In the discharge phase, in consultation with the stoma patient, all aspects that need to be taken care of before being discharged from hospital, should be checked systematically.	3
25	Ensure that the stoma care nurse is in charge of the stoma care in the postoperative phase.	3
26	Provide the stoma patient with general recommendations on healthy eating.	4
27	Ensure that the ileostomy patient, prior to discharge from the hospital, is given information by a dietician on fluid intake, nutrition and consumption of extra salt.	4
28	Ensure that the urostomy patient receives adequate advice on required fluid intake, to achieve pale yellow or straw coloured urine.	4
29	Advise the urostomy patient about the remedial benefits of cranberry juice or capsules in the event of skin- or leakage problems or (symptomatic) urinary tract infections.	3
30	Use clear, validated descriptions of the complications. Work from these valid definitions to further uniformity in nursing interventions.	3
31	Use a measuring instrument for describing and diagnosing peristomal skin disorders.	4
32	Ensure the stoma patient is aware of the symptoms related to the various potential complications or problems.	3
33	Attempt to use a stoma appliance that best suits the characteristics of the stoma, and the characteristics and personal preferences of the stoma patient.	3
34	Check regularly during three months after surgery, in consultation with the stoma patient, whether the opening of the skin barrier still fits the stoma. If necessary, adjust the stoma appliance.	4
35	Inform the stoma patient about the disposal of used stoma appliances.	4
36	In the event of complications or problems, inform the stoma patient whether a stoma care aid is indicated and, if needed and in consultation with the stoma patient, make a choice from the accessories available.	4

Chapter 6 Aftercare phase

In this chapter the specific care after discharge from hospital is described. The questions that will be answered are: "What is understood by standard stoma care in the aftercare phase?", "Complications in the aftercare phase: definitions, prevention, recognition, diagnosis and treatment" and" Choice of appliances and accessories in the aftercare phase: when to use what?"

The topics addressed are: standard stoma care in the aftercare phase, complications, choice of appliances and accessories and attention to specific patient groups.

6.1. Definition
Aftercare is the stoma management and check-ups of the stoma after the treatment. The working group states that the aftercare phase starts immediately after the patient is discharged from hospital. It is impossible to determine when this phase ends. Aftercare can be performed by the nurse in the hospital (outpatient), community nurse or community health care provider or nurses and care providers in nursing homes.

6.2. Standard stoma care in the aftercare phase
During the first period after discharge from hospital, the stoma care nurse is still the responsible co-ordinator of the stoma care. Follow-up appointments are scheduled according to a fixed schedule. If so desired, the spouse/relatives can become involved during this phase.

Ratliff et al (2005) suggest that the stoma care nurse should do the check-ups on the ostomate during the first months after discharge in the outpatient setting. In the event of complications, the stoma care nurse should increase the check-ups and assess the result of the interventions. In this phase ostomates also need education and counselling for reassurance and to support them in the proper use of the appliances.

Regarding the prevention of skin disorders, Lyon et al (2000) advise the monitoring of ostomates by a stoma care nurse before discharge from hospital and then again three months and six months after discharge. Preferably, also a check-up in the home situation in the first month after discharge from hospital should be included. Herlufsen et al (2006) advise to administer regular check-ups to prevent skin disorders, at least once a year. Claessens et al (2001) recommend, after the first year, a continuation of standard check-ups by the stoma care nurse.

Rolstad and Erwin-Toth (2010) recommend that the postoperative check-up by the stoma care nurse takes place two to four weeks after discharge, then after respectively three and six months. Annual inspections, according to Rolstad and Erwin-Toth, are part of standard care. The check-up includes inspection of skin and stoma as well as stoma appliances and accessories. The ostomate's ability to incorporate the stoma into daily life as well as the need for additional education will be assessed too.

Readding (2005) assumes that a general surgical postoperative check-up is done six weeks after discharge, and then three months thereafter. The author suggests that ostomates are unsure about follow-up appointments because they do not know what to expect. By providing proper information this can be prevented. Telephone consultation can be helpful at this stage, according to Readding.

If the ostomate has a perineum wound, it will also be checked by the stoma care nurse and she will provide information on the specific points that require attention.

In the event of a complicated wound, this is often treated multidisciplinary, i.e. in combination with a wound management nurse and/or surgeon.

It is the opinion of the working group, and this is substantiated by the findings from the literature, that the check-up visits must be performed according to a fixed schedule.

The Dutch Ostomy Association recommends that the stoma care nurse should contact the patient by telephone a few days after discharge. This enables the ostomate to immediately put forward his questions, which could prevent potential problems.

A telephone call soon after discharge reduces the ostomate's threshold to contact the stoma care nurse in the future (NSV, 2008). The stoma care nurse decides, in consultation with the ostomate, whether additional check-ups are needed. Reasons for this may be details regarding the stoma or peristomal skin or details and questions regarding the use of appliances and accessories.

The working group recommends the following schedule for the check-up visits during the first year:

1st check-up: one to two weeks after discharge (or telephone consultation).

2nd check-up: six to eight weeks after discharge.

3rd check-up: twelve to fourteen weeks after discharge.

4th check-up: nine months after discharge.

From the second year the ostomate is advised to schedule a check-up visit once a year.

Follow-up visits ideally coincide with check-ups with the responsible physician: this contributes to patient-friendliness (fewer hospital visits for the ostomate to make).

During follow-up visits the ostomate understanding of what is normal or abnormal will be assessed as well. Furthermore, tips and advice relating to day-to-day life can be given. See Appendix XV.

Recommendations: (as concluded from the abovementioned)

Recommendation 37:
Ensure that, in consultation with the ostomate, follow-up check-ups by the stoma care nurse take place.

Recommendation 38:
Schedule the check-ups at the stoma care nurse and physician simultaneously.

Recommendation 39:
Advise the ostomate to meet with the stoma care nurse for follow-up visits, starting within two weeks after discharge from hospital, thereafter every six weeks for the following three months and then after six months.

Recommendation 40:
Advise the ostomate to visit the stoma care nurse once a year, from the second year after surgery onwards, for a general stoma check-up. Adjust the care to the individual ostomate and if necessary, adjust appointment-frequency.

Conclusion level 3	
level	**Auteur title**
C	Ratliff, C.R., Scarano, K.A. & Donovan, A.M. (2005). Descriptive study of peristomal complications. *Journal of Wound Ostomy Continence Nursing, 32(1),* 33-37.
C	Herlufsen, P., Olsen, A.G., Carlsen, B., Nybaek, H., Karlsmark, T., Laursen, T.N. & Jemec, G.B.E. (2006). OstomySkin study: a study of peristomal skin disorders in patients with permanent stomas. *British Journal of Nursing, 15(16),* 854-862.
C	Claessens- Spee, C.J., Geurts, E., Kessel v, I., Vliert v/d,N., (2001). Onderzoek naar de aard en incidentie van huidproblemen bij conventionele colo, ileo en/of urinestoma. *Rondom Stomazorg, 31,* 52-57.
C	Lyon, C.C., Smith, A.J., Griffiths, C.E.M. & Beck, M.H. (2000). The spectrum of skin disorders in abdominal stoma patients. *British Journal of Dermatology, 143(6),* 1248-60.
D	Rolstad, B.S. & Erwin-Toth, P.L. (2010). Peristomal skin complications: prevention and management. *American journal of nursing, 110(2),* 43-48.
D	Readding, L.A. (2005). Hospital to home, smoothing the journey for the new ostomist. *British journal of nursing, 14(16),* 16-20.

6.2.1. Support in the home situation

In addition to contact with the stoma care nurse in the hospital, guiding and supporting the ostomate in the home situation is also important. The Dutch Ostomy Association paid working visits to self-care organizations and published a report on their findings. Only one home care institution is included in this report and some careful conclusions can be drawn from this. Since currently only a few days of hospitalization is required for stoma construction, proper guidance and counselling after discharge becomes increasingly important. In most cases a home care organization is engaged for this (NSV, 2010a).

Many ostomates are not fully independent regarding management of the stoma when discharged from hospital. In the report "Kwaliteit en organisatie van stomazorg" (NSV, 2009c) one third of the ostomates point out that they are not adequately able to take care of the stoma. The stoma care nurse or home care nurse plays an important role in teaching further self-care to the ostomate, should he be capable of participating in the learning process.

Meticulous co-ordination and exchange of knowledge and information between the hospital and home care organization is a requirement for good quality stoma care (NSV, 2010a). In the report on stoma-related complications (NSV, 2009a) a large number of ostomates indicated that no transfer was done from the hospital to the home situation or that they were not aware of this. When discharged, a complete transfer should be handed to the ostomate to allow the home care worker to continue stoma management (see Appendix XIV).

Pieper and Mikols (1996) conducted a study on the issues which worry ostomates when discharged from hospital. The two main worry-issues were fear of leakage and odour. In addition, stoma management, intimacy and sexuality and participation in sports were mentioned most frequently.

Pringle and Swan (2001) assessed 112 patients, with a colostomy due to a colorectal tumour, on how the first year after surgery progressed, and whether there had been a wish or need for nursing interventions or other medical referrals during this time. This revealed that complications such as retraction, prolapse or occurrence of parastomal hernias are the most common problems regarding the stoma in the first year. The ostomates also indicated that odour and gas forming remained a problem. The required nursing interventions all related to the need for guidance, advice on accessories and appliances, referrals to other health care providers and advice on irrigation.

Fulham (2008a) mentions that the questions that arise from the home situation differ from those during hospitalisation. Clothing, returning to work, sexuality, travelling and taking up hobbies are issues about which the ostomate may have questions or concerns.

Williams (2007) described the type of care the community nurse can offer. During the period shortly after discharge from hospital, the ostomate is particularly concerned about the appliances and accessories, possible leakage and who to turn to for help when problems arise. Wade (Williams, 2007) also indicates that most stoma problems occur in the first year after stoma construction. These problems include leakage, altered bowel pattern, retraction, prolapse, parastomal hernias and stenosis. The community nurse/care provider plays a role in identifying or detecting these problems. It is important that the ostomate is sufficiently informed about the symptoms that may occur. In addition, the community nurse or care provider can provide psycho-social support and guidance in learning to cope with the stoma. As pointed out by the Dutch Ostomy Association, most ostomates are not yet independently capable of managing their stoma when discharged from hospital. They need to be supported and in a number of cases the ostomate will never become self-supporting. This is partly influenced by physical fitness and psychological aspects. Assistance in questions such as how to incorporate the stoma into everyday life, how to deal with food, clothing, returning to work, sexuality, travelling and taking up hobbies, can also be provided by the community nurse.

Everything mentioned in Appendix VI (Discussion points preoperative counselling) may also be important in the aftercare phase.

Recommendation 41: (as concluded from abovementioned)
Discuss the home situation with the ostomate to determine whether home-support and counselling is needed to help deal with the day-to day situation. It may concern practical as well as psychosocial assistance.

Recommendation 42: (as concluded from abovementioned)
Ensure that, in consultation with the ostomate, a complete transfer is done, with the aim of guaranteeing continuity of expert stoma care.

Conclusion level 3	
level	Author title
C	Pieper, B. & Mikols, C. (1996). Predischarge and postdischarge concerns of persons with an ostomy. *Journal of wound ostomy continence nursing, 23(2)*, 105-109.
C	Pringle, W. & Swan, E. (2001). Continuing care after discharge from hospital for stoma patients. *British journal of nursing, 10(19)*, 1275-1288.

C	Nederlandse Stomavereniging (2009c). *Kwaliteit en organisatie van stomazorg. Onderzoeksverslag in opdracht van de NSV* . Amsterdam: Newcom Research & Consultancy B.V. Kapteijns, A. & Buitinga, S.
C	Nederlandse Stomavereniging (2009a). *Stomagerelateerde complicaties. Onderzoeksverslag in opdracht van de NSV* . Amsterdam: Newcom Research & Consultancy B.V. Kapteijns, A. & Buitinga, S. .
D	Nederlandse Stomavereniging (2010a). *In gesprek over de kwaliteit van de stomazorg.* Maarssen: Nederlandse Stomavereniging Eikelboom, NI.
D	Fulham, J. (2008a). A guide to caring for patients with a newly formed stoma in the acute hospital setting. *Gastrointestinal Nursing, 6(8),* 14-23.
D	Williams, J. (2007). Stoma care nursing: what the community nurse needs to know. *British journal of community nursing, 12(8),* 342- 346

6.3. Complications

As indicated in the previous chapter, the literature showed no clear distinction between possible complications in the postoperative phase and the aftercare phase (also called early and late complications). Therefore, all possible complications have been summarised in Chapter 5.

Lyon et al (2000) state that prevention and early detection of skin disorders are important because in the event of larger problems occurring, the ostomate may end up in a vicious circle: the skin disorder can cause the appliance to detach, which results in leakage and in turn prolongs the skin disorder. The risk of problems occurring is higher in ileostomy and urostomy.

Herlufsen et al (2006) did research on the incidence of skin and stoma problems. In this study, 45 percent of the participants suffered a peristomal skin disorder. Of these, 77 percent could be linked to stoma effluent. The fact that 76 percent endured these problems for more than three months is striking. Of the participants suffering skin problems, more than 80 percent did not seek professional health care.

Bosio (2007) conducted a descriptive research on peristomal disorders. One of the reasons for the study was to develop a classification model (SACS instrument). The outcome showed that skin disorders were confirmed in 52 percent of the participating ostomates.

Claessens et al (2001) studied 3166 ostomates in 77 hospitals in the Netherlands to gain insight in the incidence frequency and the nature of skin disorders. Key findings were that 40 percent of the ostomates were found to have suffered skin disorders, most commonly erythema, erosion and maceration.

The complications mentioned in the previous chapter were all validated by Colwell and Beitz. In practice however, as Claessens et al describe other complications and skin disorders encountered around the stoma, yet which are (virtually) not described in the literature and neither been validated. The most common problems are erythema (redness), maceration, erosion, stripping effect and pressure ulcers at the stoma. The working group is of the opinion that these should be mentioned here, despite incomplete support available in the literature.

In the study Claessens et al (2001) provide definitions for erythema, maceration and erosion on the accompanying scorecard. The working group formulated the definition for the stripping effect.

Complication	Definition
Erythema (redness)	change of the skin colour without further abnormalities
Maceration	Softened wet skin
Erosion	Shallow defect (abrasion) limited to the epidermis
Stripping effect	Damaged epidermis (skin) caused by frequent or careless removal of skin barrier
Pressure ulcers	Localized damage to the skin and underlying tissue, usually in the vicinity of bone protrusions, as a result of pressure or pressure in combination with friction (V&VN, Richtlijn Decubitus preventie en behandeling, 2011)

Interventions in these problems are aimed at removing or eliminating the cause, for example in the stripping effect, by adjusting the frequency or the manner of removing the skin barrier. In the case of pressure ulcers, the intervention would be to lift the pressure.

Recommendation 43: (as concluded from abovementioned)
Provide the ostomate with information about the added value of follow-up visits with regard to the prevention and incidence of stomal and peristomal problems.

Conclusion level 3	
level	Author title
C	Herlufsen, P., Olsen, A.G., Carlsen, B., Nybaek, H., Karlsmark, T., Laursen, T.N. & Jemec, G.B.E. (2006). OstomySkin study: a study of peristomal skin disorders in patients with permanent stomas. *British Journal of Nursing, 15(16),* 854-862.
C	Bosio, G. (2007). A proposal for classifying peristomal skin disorders: results of a multicenter observational study. *Ostomy Wound Manage. 53(9), 38-43.*
C	Claessens- Spee, C.J., Geurts, E., Kessel v, I., Vink, M., Vliert v/d, N., (2001). Onderzoek naar de aard en incidentie van huidproblemen bij conventionele colo, ileo en/of urinestoma. *Rondom Stomazorg, 31,* 52-57.
C	Lyon, C.C., Smith, A.J., Griffiths, C.E.M. & Beck, M.H. (2000). The spectrum of skin disorders in abdominal stoma patients. *British Journal of Dermatology, 143(6),* 1248-60.

6.4. Choice of stoma appliances

During the discharge phase, the ostomate will have made a choice regarding the stoma appliance he wants to use. Reasons for changing this choice could be incidence of complications, being unable to manage the appliance or other personal reasons, similar to those in the postoperative phase.

In connection with problems or complications, it may be necessary to change the appliance or to use other stoma accessories. The stoma care nurse should have extensive knowledge about these appliances and accessories. Using her knowledge and experience, the stoma care nurse together with the ostomate can determine whether the current appliances are correctly applied and care is carried out properly. It is then decided whether it is necessary to use other appliances and, if so, which would be suitable. In Appendix XVI, the different available appliances and accessories are listed.

In the literature, there are no criteria available regarding the number of stoma appliances to be used over a period of time. The working group considers it impossible to determine this number on a personal level, because it depends on too many different factors (as previously mentioned: stoma characteristics, patient characteristics and personal preference). It is however possible to state the average normal use for a whole group. The norm that has been applied for some time in the Netherlands is four bags per day for a colostomy, two bags per day for an ileostomy and urostomy, and four skin barriers per week for a two-piece system. If, for whatever reason the stoma appliance has to be changed more often, more appliances will be needed. In this case it is up to the expertise of the stoma care nurse to assess together with the ostomate, if different stoma appliances or a different approach could help reduce the frequency of care and consequently reduce appliance consumption.

Recommendation 44: (as concluded from abovementioned)
Ensure as a stoma care nurse, to have knowledge of all available stoma accessories and aids and their applicability.

Recommendation 45: (as concluded from abovementioned)
In the event of complications or other problems, inform the ostomate about other available stoma accessories. In consultation with the ostomate, supported by the the expertise of the stoma care nurse, make a selection from the available materials.

6.5. Stoma irrigation

In this phase, the ostomate (with a colostomy) can choose to irrigate. Irrigation means to flush the colon on a regular basis with the help of special accessories so that the ostomate will be free from faecal discharges for 24 up to 48 hours. Colostomy irrigation has been a management option since the 1920's (Turnbull, 2003). The reasons for irrigation are diverse. It gives the ostomate a feeling of continence and if skin disorders are caused by leakage of faeces onto the skin, these disorders are reduced. The stoma can then be managed with a stoma patch, mini bag or plug. Disadvantages are that the irrigation process is time consuming and there is a possibility of physical reactions due to flushing with water. Risk of bowel perforation can also be regarded as a disadvantage, however, by using a cone rather than a catheter, this risk is minimal (Barr, 2004; Erwin-Toth, 2006).
Irrigation is only possible in a colostomy. Before the ostomate can be instructed on irrigation by a stoma care nurse, permission must be asked from the physician. Important aspects that should be considered are the length and function of the remaining intestine and other physical problems such as the presence of a parastomal hernia or cardiovascular problems. The stoma care nurse also discusses with the ostomate if there are other concerns such as limited dexterity, vision, cognitive aspects, etc. In addition, the home situation must be sufficient suitable (adequate toilet space should be available for the time needed to irrigate).
Karadag et al (2004) did research on the relationship between quality of life and irrigation. The conclusion was that under certain circumstances irrigation proves to be a safe method to obtain continence and can contribute to improving quality of life in specific areas.

Recommendation 46: (as concluded from abovementioned)
After consultation with the physician, inform the ostomate about the possibility of irrigation. Ensure that the instruction is done by the stoma care nurse. The amount of water used during, the frequency of, and the time required for flushing, differs for each person.

Conclusion level 3	
level	Author title
B	Karadaĝ, A., Menteş, B.B., & Ayaz, S. (2004). Colostomy Irrigation: results of 25 cases with particular reference to quality of life. *Journal of Clinical Nursing, 14(4)*, 479-485.
C	Karadaĝ, A., Menteş, B.B., Üner, A., İrKörücü, O., Ayaz, S. & Özkan, S. (2003). Impact of stomatherapy in quality of life in patients with permanent colostomies or ileostomies. *International Journal of Colorectal Disease, 18(3)*, 234-238.
D	Turnbull, GB (2003). A look at the purpose and outcomes of colostomy irrigation. *Ostomy wound management, 49(2)*, 19-20.

Recommendation 47: (as concluded from the abovementioned)
Advise to use a cone rather than a catheter for irrigation.

Conclusion level 4	
level	Author title
D	Barr, JE (2004). Assessment and management of stomal complications: a framework for clinical decision making. *Stoma care wound manage. 50(9)*, 50- 67.
D	Erwin-Toth, P., (2006). Ostomy care and rehabilitation in colorectal cancer. *Seminars in oncology nursing, 22(3)*, 174-177.

6. 6. Specific patient groups

No clinical question was formulated with regard to specific groups, however, it was decided to dedicate a paragraph to this group consisting of pregnant women and obese patients. Both have been discussed in a number of articles. The working group considers the issues that came to light in these articles as sufficiently important and therefore included them in this guideline. Due to the increase of the abdomen and hormonal changes during pregnancy, extra attention is needed in the stoma care.

Given the expected increase of obese patients, it was decided to address this group of patients in the guideline as well. As mentioned, many articles describe risks or other issues related to obese patients with a stoma, all of which may require attention.

6. 6 .1. Pregnancy

Aukamp and Sredle have published joint publications on pregnant women and stoma. Pregnancy does not necessarily have to be problematic to the stoma. However, there are additional issues that need attention. Due to the enlarged abdomen, adjustments of stoma appliances are required. The stoma may increase in size or retract. Due to overall improved blood circulation during pregnancy, the stoma might also have better blood supply. Hormonal changes may affect the skin.

Additional nursing interventions may be needed with regard to adjusting the opening of the skin barrier and exchanging materials such as the convex skin barrier with more flexible material. In addition extra advice, such as the use of a mirror for improved stoma visibility, may be required or helpful.

Problems or complications that would normally occur can be aggravated by the pregnancy. Complications may include: dehydration and disturbed electrolyte balance caused by nausea and vomiting, urinary tract infection, obstipation and obstruction. In addition, there can be an increase of parastomal hernia, bleeding, retraction, stenosis, damage to the stoma or pain around the stoma (particularly postpartum). Excessive vomiting can cause a hernia or prolapse. Despite these complications, pregnant women with a stoma can have a normal pregnancy, childbirth and postpartum period. Ostomates can use a support bandage to support the abdominal wall. Caesarean section may be required in case of obstruction, but is usually only performed for obstetric reasons. The authors recommend that close co-operation between the obstetrician and the stoma care nurse is ensured (Aukamp and Sredle, 2004; Sredle and Aukamp, 2006).

Recommendation 48: (as concluded from the abovementioned)
Advise the ostomate to stay under supervision of a stoma care nurse during pregnancy, because adjustments of the stoma appliance and additional counselling may be needed.

Recommendation 49: (as concluded from the abovementioned)
If necessary, contact the midwife or obstetrician.

Conclusion level 4	
level	**Author title**
D	Aukamp, V. & Sredl, D. (2004) Collaborative care management for a pregnant woman with an ostomy. *Complementary therapy in nursing & midwifery, 10(1)*, 5-12.
D	Sredl, D. & Aukamp, V. (2006). Evidence-based nursing care management for the pregnant women with an ostomy. *Journal of wound ostomy continence nursing, 33(1)*, 42-49.

6.6.2. Obesity

Park et al (1999) conducted studies on stoma complications, and found no correlation between a high BMI and stoma complications.

Aramugan et al (2002) investigated stoma complications and the risk factors for complications. The results of their study showed that a high BMI is a significant risk factor for the development of retraction, erosive skin damage and leakage.

Kouba et al (2007) studied the occurrence of complications in urostomy for the duration of at least one year after surgery. The study showed that the incidence of complications in two groups with a BMI > 25 and a BMI > 30, was higher than in the group with a BMI < 25. In addition, this study showed that the combination of a higher BMI and older age increases the risk of complications.

A study by De Raet et al (2008) looked at the risk factors for parastomal hernia after an abdominal perineal resection. This showed that a waist circumference of more than 100 cm is a significant risk factor for the development of a parastomal hernia.

A small study done by Richebourg et al (2007) indicates that ostomates with a higher BMI have a shorter wear time of the stoma appliances. Ostomates with a normal BMI (18.5 -24.9) mention an average wear time of four days and those with a BMI > 30 , a wear time of 3,2 days.

Recommendation 50: (as concluded from the abovementioned)
For obese ostomates additional information should be provided and extra check-ups are required due to the increased risk of physical problems and complications.

Conclusion level 3	
level	**Author title**
C	Arumugam, P.J., Bevan, L., Macdonald, L., Watkins, A.J., Morgan, A.R., Beynon, J. & Carr, N.D. (2003). A prospective audit of stoma analysis of risk factors and complications. *Colorectal Disease, 5(1),* 49-52.
C	Park, J.J., Del Pino, A., Orsay, C.P., Nelson, R.L., Pearl, L.K., Cintron, J.R. & Abcarian, H. (1999). Stoma complications: the Cook County Hospital experience. *Diseases of the Colon & Rectum, 42(12),* 1575-1580.
C	Kouba, E., Sands, M., Lentz, A., Wallen, E. & Pruthi, R.S. (2007). Incidence and Risk Factors of stomal complications in patients undergoing cystectomy with ileal conduit urinary diversion for bladder cancer. *The Journal of Urology, 178(3),* 950-954
C	Richbourg, L., Thorpe, J.M. & Rapp, C.G. (2007). Difficulties experienced by the ostomate after hospital discharge. *Journal of Wound Ostomy Continence Nursing, 34 (1) ,* 70-79.
C	De Raet, J., Delvaux, G., Haentjens, P. & Van Nieuwenhove, Y. (2008). Waist circumference is an independent risk factor for the development of parastomal hernia after permanent colostomy. *Diseases of the Colon & Rectum, 51(12),* 1806–09

Duchesne et al (2002) indicate that obese patients have a higher risk of suffering postoperative complications and it is recommended to pay extra attention to this during counselling and education. Stoma siting also needs more attention, possibly in consultation with the surgeon (also see paragraph 4.2.B.1.).
Gallagher and Gates (2004) describe the issues in obese patients with a stoma. They state that these ostomates have a higher risk of problems occurring and it is therefore likely that they need more help. Involving relatives is therefore even more important. In addition, Gallagher and Gates, as well as Vink (2007) plead for a multidisciplinary approach specifically aimed at this patient group.
Vink (2007) mentions issues relating to the care of the stoma. If the stoma is less accessible to the ostomate, emptying the stoma bag or changing the appliance can be problematic.
Colwell and Fichera (2005) describe the advice to be given to ostomates with a high BMI who need a re-operation in connection with a parastomal hernia: they should lose weight prior to surgery. For this, guidance is required.

Recommendation 51: (as concluded from the abovementioned)
Involve relatives of obese patients since there is a chance the obese patient will require more assistance due to the increased risk of physical problems and complications.

Conclusion level 3	
level	Author title
B	Duchesne, J.C., Wang, Y.Z., Weintraub, S.L., Boyle, M. & Hunt, J.P. (2002). Stoma complications: a multivariate analysis. *The American Surgeon, 68(11),* 961-968.
D	Gallagher, S. & Gates, J. (2004).Challenges of ostomy care and obesity. O*stomy wound management, 50(9),* 38-46.
D	Colwell, J.C. & Fichera, A. (2005). Care of the obese patient with an ostomy. *Journal of Wound Stoma care Continence Nursing, 32(6)*, 378-383.
D	Vink, M. (2007). De obese patiënte en stomazorg. *WCS nieuws, 24(1),* 45-47.

	Recommendation	Conclusion level
37	Ensure that, in consultation with the ostomate, follow-up check-ups by the stoma care nurse take place.	3
38	Schedule the check-ups at the stoma care nurse and physician simultaneously.	3
39	Advise the ostomate to meet with the stoma care nurse for follow-up visits, starting within two weeks after discharge from hospital, thereafter every six weeks for the following three months and then after six months.	3
40	Advise the ostomate to visit the stoma care nurse once a year, from the second year after surgery onwards, for a general stoma check-up. Adjust the care to the individual ostomate and if necessary, adjust appointment-frequency.	3
41	Discuss the home situation with the ostomate to determine whether home-support and -counselling is needed to help deal with the day-to day situation. It may concern practical as well as psychosocial assistance.	3
42	Ensure that, in consultation with the ostomate, a complete transfer is done, with the aim of guaranteeing continuity of expert stoma care.	3
43	Provide the ostomate with information about the added value of follow-up visits with regard to the prevention and incidence of stomal and peristomal problems.	3
44	Ensure as a stoma care nurse, to have knowledge of all available stoma accessories and aids and their applicability.	4
45	In the event of complications or other problems, inform the ostomate about other available stoma accessories. In consultation with the ostomate, supported by the expertise of the stoma care nurse, make a selection from the available materials.	4
46	After consultation with the physician, inform the ostomate about the possibility of irrigation. Ensure that the instruction is done by the stoma care nurse. The amount of water used during, the frequency of, and the time required for flushing, differs for each person.	3
47	Advise to use a cone rather than a catheter for irrigation.	4
48	Advise the ostomate to stay under supervision of a stoma care nurse during pregnancy, because adjustments of the stoma appliance and additional counselling may be needed.	4
49	If necessary, contact the midwife or obstetrician.	4
50	For obese ostomates additional information should be provided and extra check-ups are required due to the increased risk of physical problems and complications.	3
51	Involve relatives of obese patients since there is a chance the obese patient will require more assistance due to the increased risk of physical problems and complications.	4

Chapter 7 Organizing stoma care

This chapter focuses on the requirements of organizing stoma care in the Netherlands in such a way that the recommendations in this guideline can be implemented.

The questions that will be answered are: "Which care provider performs what care and when; what level of expertise is required?", "Which continuity of care is required" and "Which disciplines are involved in the stoma care?"

Unlike in previous chapters, where the recommendations relate to the content of stoma care, the recommendations in this chapter relate to policy and organizing the stoma care.

In order to provide proper stoma care to patients throughout the entire process, several conditions must be met. With regard to organizing stoma care, three aspects are distinguished:
The care process: providing insight in the steps of the process the patient goes through.
Care providers: what level of expertise and what disciplines are involved? Who can perform which tasks?
Logistical conditions: consulting or working space and set-up, time, materials, brochures, etc.

7. 1. The care process

The following pages include a flow chart of the care process. The chart makes the care process transparent and links are made to points in the process where the (stoma) nurse plays a role. The care process is broken down into two phases: the clinical phase and the phase after discharge from hospital (outpatient or in the home situation). This care chart dictates the process the (future) ostomate has to follow from the moment it becomes known that he (may) receive a stoma. The stages of this process (preoperative phase, clinical, postoperative phase and the aftercare phase) are used in this guideline to answers the questions as formulated in chapter one. In the event of an emergency situation or when the stoma has to be constructed unexpectedly, some aspects are moved from the preoperative to the postoperative phase. The care provider is aware of the contents of the care chart.

Patient's care process from registration till clinical discharge

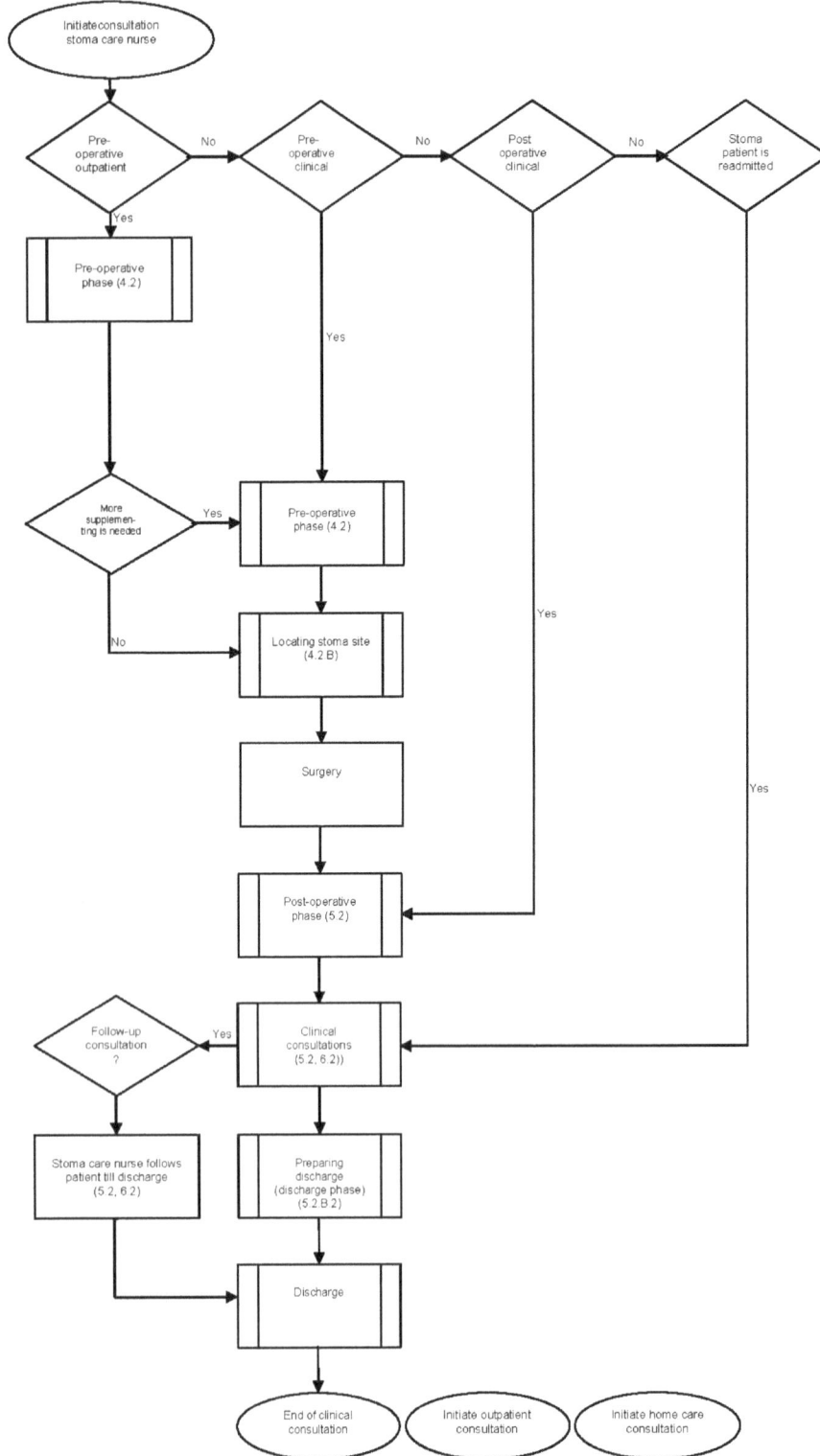

Ostomate's care process after discharge in the outpatient setting

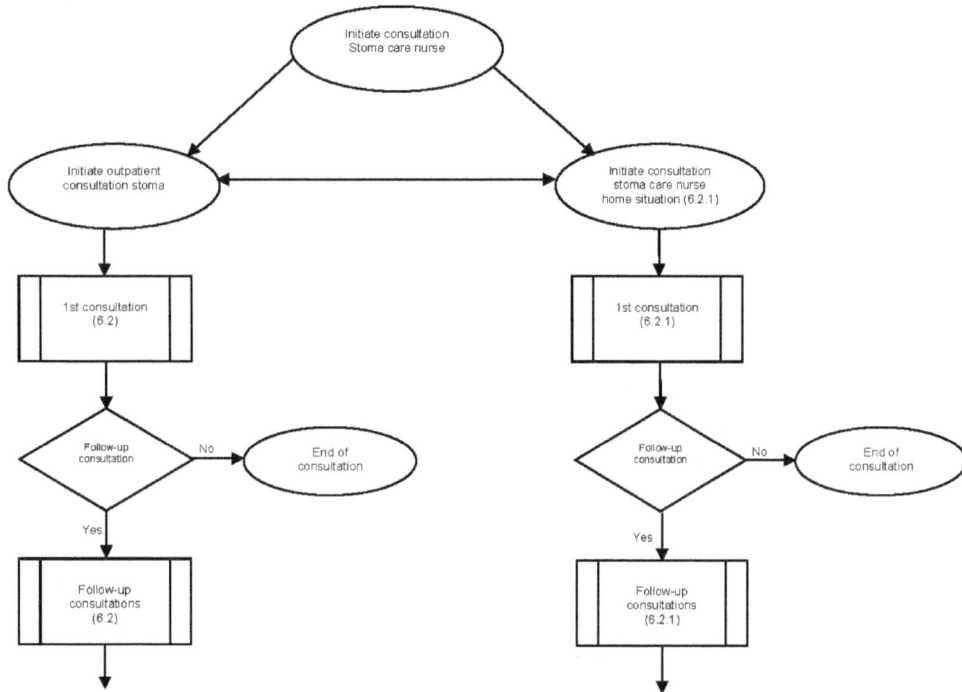

Explanation of the symbols used in the flow chart

Symbol		
(oval)	Signals the beginning or end of a process	Shows the beginning or end of a process
(pre-established process)	Pre-established process	Indicates steps in the process that are described elsewhere. Often used in cases with sub-processes
(diamond)	Decision-making moment	Presents a question which can be answered with yes or no
(rectangle)	Process or activity	Shows a process or action

7.2. The health care providers

The ostomate may be faced with many different health care professionals, medical as well as nursing or caring.

Within the group of nurses and care providers involved in ostomy there is a differentiation with respect to the function level. As described in the "BIG"-law, care providers must be qualified and consider themselves capable of performing certain tasks. This too applies to the procedures related to the ostomate. Whether a nurse or care provider can be employed to perform stoma care tasks depends mainly on their competence. This means that the nurse or care provider should possess the (theoretical) knowledge and skills required by the function, and a correct attitude towards the ostomate.

The V&VN Department of Stoma Care Nurses wrote an occupational profile for the stoma care nurse in 2004. This profile was updated in 2009. In addition, new general occupational profiles were released in March 2012 by the V&VN, however discussion of these topics is beyond the scope and time frame of this guideline.

To determine the competencies that are needed within the ostomy, organizations are advised to consult the documents mentioned above.

7.2.1. Skills levels of nurses and care providers

Different (nursing) tasks within the ostomy have different degrees of complexity. In Appendix XVII the specific tasks are listed as well as the related level of competence which, according to the working group, is required. It is assumed that every nurse or care provider is aware of her own competences in order to determine if she is able to provide support and care herself or whether the ostomate should be referred to other health care professionals.

Uncomplicated ostomy can be performed by nurses and care providers of level three IG. 'Uncomplicated care' means the changing of stoma appliances (skin barrier and bag) in the absence of skin disorders, stoma problems or other factors that may affect the care of the stoma. It is important that the care provider is able to, and subsequently recognizes a stoma problem or skin disorder, or any other changes that may occur, and responds adequately. 'Responding adequately' means to enlist the help of a care professional with more knowledge and experience regarding ostomy, who is able to determine the appropriate interventions and possible implementation. Problems that are not recognized or managed in time, can lead to even greater problems.

In the outpatient setting as well as in hospitals there are nurses who perform stoma care as part of their regular nursing job, but who also received advanced follow-up training in ostomy. Immediate colleagues can turn to these nurses with their questions on ostomy. In the event a specialist stoma care nurse is not available, these particular nurses can temporarily fill in for them.

However, in the event of specific problems, complications, questions relating to use or change of appliances/accessories, or in the case of highly complex issues, the ostomate should always be referred to a stoma care nurse.

Recommendation 52: (as concluded from the abovementioned)
Adjust the level of job-competence to the complexity of the care. Uncomplicated stoma care can be executed from level three IG. In the case of abnormal situations or complications a level four or five-nurse should be allocated to the patient.

Recommendation 53: (as concluded from the abovementioned)
Refer the ostomate to the stoma care nurse in the event of complications.

7.2.2. Level of expertise of nurses and care providers

A literature review was done to answer the question about the level of expertise required to ensure proper stoma care. Several studies explored the relationship between quality of (general) care and the level of education and experience of care providers.

The study by Needleman et al (2002) indicated that there are fewer complications and shorter hospital stay in cases where highly educated nurses were involved in stoma care during longer hours.

Aiken et al (2003) also investigated the relationship between education of nurses and the number of complications. They conclude that a larger number of higher educated nurses yield a lower mortality rate and occurrence of "failure to rescue" (death after complications).

Blegen et al (2001) looked into the relationship between the level of training and increase in the quality of care, which is measured based on the incidence of patient's falling and medication errors made. The conclusion of this study is that there is no link between a higher level of education and fewer medication errors or falls. The outcome of the care however, is noticeably better because of the presence of experienced nurses.

Kendall - Gallagher et al (2011) specifically investigated the effects of specialised nursing care on the outcomes of the care. They conclude that specialised nursing care is associated with better care outcomes. The authors have found no evidence for better results due to specialised care alone. The combination of specialised care with higher education seems to result in better care outcomes. They therefore argue that increasing the overall education level will be more beneficial to hospitals and patients than specifically training the lower skilled nurses.

Since all these studies have been conducted in the United States (with a different skills level set-up than in the Netherlands), a transcription to the exact level of education in the Netherlands (level four, five or Nursing Specialist) is not available.

Recommendation 54: (as concluded from the abovementioned)
Ensure that there are sufficient trained nurses available to achieve good care outcomes.

Conclusion level 2	
level	Author title
B	Needleman, J., Buerhaus, P., Mattke, S., Stewart, M. & Zelevinsky, K., (2002). Nurse staffing levels and the quality of care in hospitals. *The New England Journal of Medicine. 346(22,)* 1715-22. Verkregen op 10-8-2012 nejm.org
B	Aiken, L.H., Clarke, S.P., Cheung, R.B., Sloane D.M. & Silber, J.H. (2003). Educational levels of hospital nurses and surgical patient mortality. *JAMA. 290(12),* 1617- 23.

B	Kendall- Gallagher, D., Aiken, L.H., Sloane, D.M. & Cimiotti J.P. (2011). Nurse specialty certification, inpatient mortality, and failure to rescue. *Journal of Nursing scholarship, 43(2), 188-194.*
B	Blegen, M.A., Vaughn, T.E. & Goode, C.J. (2001). Nurse Experience and Education: Effect on Quality of Care. *The Journal of Nursing Administration, 31(1)*, 33-39.

7.2.3. Other specialist care providers

In addition to nurses and care providers, the ostomate will also have to deal with various other (medical) care professionals, such as: a gastroenterologist, a (gastro-intestinal) surgeon, a urologist, a dermatologist, an oncologist and a GP. He can even be referred to a sexologist, a psychologist or a social worker. In many cases, a dietician is engaged and sometimes a physical therapist. In addition to the stoma care nurse other specialised nurses such as a colon care/MDL nurse, an oncology nurse or a wound management nurse may be involved.

Although many different health care professionals are involved in an ostomate or stoma patients' care, the stoma care nurse is responsible for co-ordinating the multidisciplinary treatment and care of the stoma. As case manager, the stoma care nurse will therefore have to promote good multidisciplinary co-operation between all parties involved.

Recommendation 55: (as concluded from the abovementioned)
Ensure that the stoma care nurse acts as a case manager, in order to promote multidisciplinary co-operation between all the care professionals involved.

7.3. The task of the stoma care nurse

Both the Dutch Ostomy Association (2009c) and the Dutch Society of Surgery (NVvH) plead for the presence of a stoma care nurse in hospitals (and community home care) where stoma care is provided.

The standards for surgical treatments (NVvH, 2011) state that hospitals where colon cancer is treated "have a stoma clinic and stoma care nurse or nurse trained in the ostomy at hand". The working group expects that the organisational conditions for such personnel are met as mentioned in the introduction to this chapter.

The RNAO (2009) also recommends that a stoma care nurse should be available and be facilitated, amongst others, for the development of policy.

Recommendation 56: (as concluded from the abovementioned)
Ensure that a stoma care nurse is employed in each institution where stoma care is offered. These institutions should facilitate the stoma care nurses.

Conclusion level 3	
level	**Author title**
C	Nederlandse Stomavereniging (2009c). *Kwaliteit en organisatie van stomazorg. Onderzoeksverslag in opdracht van de NSV.* Amsterdam: Newcom Research & Consultancy B.V. Kapteijns, A. & Buitinga, S.
D	Nederlandse Vereniging voor Heelkunde (2011). Normen voor chirurgische behandeling. Verkregen op 31-3-2012 <<*www.kwaliteitskoepel.nl/assets/structured-files/Normen/*>>

AGREE	Registered nurses' association of Ontario. (2009). *Ostomy care and management. Clinical best practice guidelines*. Ontario: RNAO. Verkregen op 14-2-2011 www.rnao.org/bestpractices

7.3.1. Added value of the stoma care nurse

Apart from the general level of education, the literature was searched for evidence on the added value of the input of the stoma care nurse. Apart from the differentiation in level of competence, it is also possible to describe a differentiation with respect to content. The stoma care nurse is a BIG-registered nurse with a specialization. Sometimes hospitals differentiate between stoma care nurses in the clinic or in the outpatient setting on the one hand, and stoma care nurses specifically employed for colostomy or urostomy.

The importance of a specialised stoma care nurse is shown in several studies.

A study by Millan (2009) shows the importance of stoma care in the preoperative phase. A group of patients with preoperative stoma support was compared to a group that had received no support. The group with stoma care support experienced significantly less stoma complications and indicated to having suffered less from anxiety.

In the review by Brown and Randle (2004) Baxter and Salter (2000) state that stoma care nurses can play a key role in caring for patients with a stoma, both pre- and postoperatively. They identify ways in which nurses can help stoma patients: helping the patients come to terms with their diagnosis and prognosis; adapting to life with a stoma; teaching practical skills in stoma management; contact with relatives and friends with relation to the stoma; body image and sexuality.

In their conclusion Brown and Randle state that the stoma care nurse is responsible for monitoring the process of the stoma patient. Due to her function, the stoma care nurse is in the perfect position for safeguarding continuity of care. And because of her position, the patients can express their concerns and problems to her and she can support every individual patient. This review also states that the nurse specialist can focus on a clearly defined area of clinical practice as a result of additional training and specific experience. Specialised stoma care nurses base their practice on evidence (Brown and Randle, 2004).

Wu et al (2007) conclude that the nurse pays attention to the ostomate's needs and the impact of the stoma on social life. Wu et al also state that the stoma care nurse has a role in providing general information on a stoma. This may prevent prejudice and discrimination and create an open atmosphere regarding stoma in general. In addition, Wu et al indicate that the stoma care nurse has a role in the development of stoma care and planning interventions so that patients and their families can learn to cope with a stoma (become empowered).

Pringle and Swan (2001) examined patients with a colostomy as a result of a colorectal tumour, in order to determine the progress in the first year after surgery and whether there was a necessity or need for nursing interventions or referral. The study shows the importance of guiding ostomates during home visits after discharge from hospital. The stoma care nurse can identify problems and complications and if necessary, refer the patient or provide counselling and support.

In the review of Butler (2009), the role of the stoma care nurse in the different phases is described. In the preoperative phase, the importance of the stoma care nurse is emphasized in preoperative counselling and in locating the stoma site. In the postoperative phase the stoma care nurse is responsible for observation and functioning of the stoma, using suitable stoma materials and preventing complications. Butler (and Duchesne, 2002) furthermore state that fast recognition and intervention are necessary for optimal treatment of the complications. The purpose of the stoma care nurse is to help the ostomate to adapt to life with a stoma (Butler, 2009).

Ratliff et al (2005) assessed ostomates for the presence of peristomal complications when they returned for their 2-month postoperative check-up. The measuring instrument was developed from categories derived from the WOCN guideline and the interrater reliability of this instrument had been tested by users. One of the conclusions is that due to shorter hospital stays, less time is available for learning stoma management and learning to solve (skin) problems. Patients need more education and follow-up after discharge in order to be confident about caring for the stoma and using stoma material. It offers a challenge to the stoma care nurse to achieve this within the given situation.

The EAUN (2009) also recommends ostomates to always have access to a stoma care nurse. These findings are supported by the research of the Dutch Ostomy Association: ostomates were asked whether the stoma care nurse had added value. Virtually all the ostomates (91 percent) considered the stoma care nurse to have added value (NSV, 2009c).

Recommendation 57: (as concluded from the abovementioned)
Make sure that the ostomate has access to a stoma care nurse.

Conclusion level 2	
level	Author title
B	Millan, M. (2009) Preoperative stoma siting and education by stomatherapists of colorectal cancer patients: a descriptive study in twelve Spanish colorectal units. *Colorectal disease, 12,* 88-92.
B	Brown, H. & Randle, J. (2005). Living with a stoma: a review of the literature. *Journal of clinical nursing, 14,* 74-81.
B	Duchesne, J.C., Wang, Y.Z., Weintraub, S.L., Boyle, M. & Hunt, J.P. (2002). Stoma complications: a multivariate analysis. *The American Surgeon, 68(11),* 961-968.
C	Wu, H.K.M., Chau, J.P.C. & Twinn, S., (2007). Self-efficacy and quality of life among stoma patients in Hong Kong. *Cancer Nursing, 30(3),* 186-193.
C	Pringle, W. & Swan, E. (2001). Continuing care after discharge from hospital for stoma patients. *British journal of nursing, 10(19),* 1275-1288.
C	Butler, D.L.(2009). Early postoperative complications following ostomy surgery: a review. *Journal of wound ostomy continence nursing, 36(5),* 513-519.
C	Ratliff, C.R., Scarano, K.A., Donovan, A.M. (2005). Descriptive study of peristomal complications. *Journal of wound ostomy continence nursing, 32(1),* 33-37.
C	Nederlandse Stomavereniging (2009c). *Kwaliteit en organisatie van stomazorg. Onderzoeksverslag in opdracht van de NSV.* Amsterdam: Newcom Research & Consultancy B.V. Kapteijns, A. & Buitinga, S.
AGREE	European Association of Urology Nurses (2009). *Good practice in health care: incontinent urostomy.* European Association of Urology Nurses Geng, V., Cobussen, H., Fillingham, S., Holroyd, S., Kiesbye, B. & Vahr, S.

7.3.2. The task of the stoma care nurse in community care

Most hospitals employ a stoma care nurse and various community care organizations have stoma care nurses on their staff. In the previously mentioned report of the Dutch Ostomy Association (NSV, 2010a), attention is also paid to the task of the stoma care nurse in community care. The presence of a stoma care nurse in the outpatient setting offers many advantages for both the ostomate and community health care personnel. The lines of communication between the stoma care nurse and the community health care workers are kept short, allowing for resolving and prevention of problems in an early stage. The stoma care nurse will, if necessary, make house calls and subsequently play a role in spreading practical knowledge and information on stomata and stoma care and in providing other forms of support. Good quality of care is enhanced by the close contacts which usually exist between stoma care nurses in community care institutions and those at the hospital. This also allows for better continuity of care.

Several community care institutions send a stoma care nurse to nursing homes or care homes to visit ostomates for a consultation.

The stoma care nurse can also play a role in enhancing community care workers' and nursing home staff's expertise (NSV, 2010a).

Recommendation 58: (as concluded from the abovementioned)
Promote the continuity of stoma care in the home situation by employing a stoma care nurse in the outpatient setting.

Conclusion level 4	
level	Author title
D	Nederlandse Stomavereniging (2010a). *In gesprek over de kwaliteit van de stomazorg.* Maarssen: Nederlandse Stomavereniging Eikelboom, N.I.

7.3.3. Training, experience and responsibilities of the stoma care nurse

Stoma care nurses are BIG-registered generic nurses who followed advanced training in ostomy. The Netherlands offers various trainings on different levels. Besides the theoretical training, practical training is indispensable. In the way the surgical professional group sets standards with respect to the number of surgical procedures to be performed each year (experience requirement), standards with regard to required practical experience could be set for stoma care nurses. To date, there is no minimum requirement set by the professional group for neither theoretical nor practical experience. The stoma care nurse is given the possibility for registration in the V&VN quality register.

After the follow-up training, the stoma care nurse will have to stay informed on the development within the ostomy by e.g. attending symposia, visiting (inter)national conferences and reading publications. It is also important they follow research and development on stoma appliances and materials.

Recommendation 59: (as concluded from the abovementioned)
Ensure as a stoma care nurse to get sufficient training and practical experience and stay well informed on developments within the field of ostomy care.

Recommendation 60: (as concluded from the abovementioned)
Ensure as a stoma care nurse registration in the V&VN quality register and the subregister of ostomy care.

Tasks and job description of the stoma care nurse
Klok (2006) inventoried Dutch stoma care nurses' functions. The specific tasks that were regarded as part of the function of the stoma care nurse were also included.
Following is an incomplete list of specific tasks related to ostomy as mentioned by the participants in this inventory:
Preoperative consultation, siting, choice of materials for discharge, treating skin disorders and/or stoma complications and advice in high-output. Postoperative consultation after emergency surgery, instruction of the patient (with spouse and/or relatives), removing sutures, removing bridge, ordering materials for discharge, advising and/or treating obstruction.
All these tasks can be performed by the stoma care nurse but she can also have a co-ordinating role in this.

The following list, formulated by the working group, gives a more general description of the contents of the function of the stoma care nurse.
• Role of an expert/consultation/active role in multidisciplinary consultation
• Promoting level of expertise of the disciplines involved
• Quality of care: developing protocols, developing policy
• Innovation, research
• Management of materials
• Organizing the stoma clinic and stoma care within the organization
• Function development, public relations
• Keep up own expertise level (theoretical knowledge and knowledge on stoma materials and aids)
It is beyond the scope of this guideline to include a complete job description. This list is aimed to give a general impression of the tasks and job description of the stoma care nurse. The stoma care nurse has an independent function, and it may be expected that she can actively put this into practice.

7. 4. Logistical conditions
The reasons for employing a stoma care nurse in every organization where stoma care is provided to ostomates has been substantiated in the paragraphs above. A number of logistical conditions like office space and equipment, time and a variety of materials should be in place to enable the stoma nurse to perform her tasks.

The following applies to the stoma care nurse at the hospital as well as in community care, except for the workspace where direct patient care is performed (in most cases this would be the home of the ostomate). This paragraph briefly describes the logistical requirements needed for the stoma care nurse to provide high quality of care.

Workspace
A furnished consultation room should be available. This space must be suitable for the following tasks: consultation, assessment/treatment/care of the stoma, instruction and administrative work. Space for storage of materials is also required.
During consultations with (potential) ostomates, brochures and other educational tools are used. These items should be available in the same room or somewhere in the vicinity. This also applies for computers for multimedia information.
A consultation room is needed for assessment, treatment and care of the stoma, as well as for storage of stoma materials and aids. In addition, the room is used for giving instruction or teaching how to irrigate and should have direct access to a toilet.
It is preferred that this workspace is located in the vicinity of the other care providers involved in ostomy care.
To enable patient administration, access to patient files is needed (a computer connected to the hospital system or paper files).

Materials
With regard to materials the stoma care nurse must have access to a wide range of stoma materials of assorted brands, models and designs. It is also necessary that the various existing ostomy appliances are at hand. This is to enable immediate intervention when stomal or peristomal problems have been identified and to instruct the use of these materials.
Other materials are the various information brochures, books and multimedia. Computers are needed for several reasons: patient administration, counselling, development of educational programs, quality and training.

7.4.1. Staffing
The second aspect of the inventory of Klok (2006) concerns the number of full-time equivalent (FTE). In this inventory, respondents were asked about the number of hours available for stoma care in relation to the supply of new stoma patients. In this survey, data from 40 hospitals was processed. In 20 hospitals the respondents regarded the time available as sufficient and in the 20 other hospitals the time was considered insufficient. A striking finding was that there appears to be a connection between the number of check-ups performed and the supply of new stoma patients. In the clinical phase, stoma care nurses meet, on average, four times with stoma patients. In hospitals with up to fifty new patients the average is six times. However, in hospitals with more than 200 new patients, an average of only two times per admission is reached. A similar trend is seen in the follow-up visits. The average is four visits in the first year. When the number of new ostomates per year drops, the average of follow-up visits increase to six per year. However, when the number of new ostomates per year, reach 150 or more, the visits are

down to two or three per year. It seems that the number of check-ups during admission and follow-up visits is determined by the time available and not by quality criteria in place. Data analysis from this survey shows that "the turning point at which the available hours are no longer experienced as sufficient, is between 90 and 100 new patients per FTE per year".

The required staffing is also influenced by the developments in health care. Without additional research it is therefore impossible to deduce that, for example in the case where a shift from clinical to outpatient care was made, more of less staff is required.

The working group recommends the development of a staffing guideline for ostomy. Using the above-mentioned inventory, the working group proposes that:

Based on Klok's inventory and practical experiences of the members of the group, 1 FTE (for a stoma care nurse) per 90 new stoma patients per year is required to ensure quality of stoma care, as recommended in this guideline, is made possible. (Provided that 1FTE equals 36 hours per week.) The preceding items are also in the interest of the extramural stoma care.

Nr.	level	Author title
313	D	Klok, S.I. (2006). Uitwerking enquête raamwerk functie stomaverpleegkundige. *Rondom Stomazorg, 19(40)*, 16-17.

	Recommendation	Conclusion level
52	Adjust the level of job-competence to the complexity of the care. Uncomplicated stoma care can be executed from level three IG. In the case of abnormal situations or complications a level four or five nurse should be allocated to the patient.	4
53	Refer the ostomate to the stoma care nurse in the event of complications.	4
54	Ensure that there are sufficient trained nurses available to achieve good care outcomes.	2
55	Ensure that the stoma care nurse acts as a case manager, in order to promote multidisciplinary co-operation between all the care professionals involved.	4
56	Ensure that a stoma care nurse is employed in each institution where stoma care is offered. These institutions should facilitate the stoma care nurses.	3
57	Make sure that the ostomate has access to a stoma care nurse.	2
58	Promote the continuity of stoma care in the home situation by employing a stoma care nurse in the outpatient setting.	4
59	Ensure as a stoma care nurse to get sufficient training and practical experience and stay well informed on developments within the field of ostomy care.	4
60	Ensure as a stoma care nurse registration in the V&VN quality register and the subregister of ostomy care.	4

Chapter 8
Accountability, implementation, evaluation and assessment

8.1. Accountability
This guideline was developed for nurses and care providers involved in stoma care. The document was compiled on the evidence available at the time of writing. It is subject to new scientific insights which may develop in the course of time.

In drafting the guideline uses the input from a sounding board, consisting of members of the Dutch Ostomy Association, the Dutch Association of Dieticians, Dutch Association of Urology, Dutch Association of Dermatology and Venereology, the Dutch Association of Surgery and the Dutch Association of Gastroenterologists. The members of the sounding board were acting on behalf of their respective associations. Hanny Cobussen-Boekhorst supplied advice in her individual capacity.

In accordance with the script for the development of this guideline on ostomy, the concept was published on the website of the Association of Nurses and Care providers in the Netherlands (V&VN), Department of Stoma Care Nurses, and its members were given the opportunity to respond. During the V&VN annual meeting in 2012 the guideline was accepted with a majority of votes.

The working group members declare that they have no conflicting interests with regard to the contents of this guideline.

8.2. Dissemination (distribution)
The guideline is available in Dutch as a pdf-file on the website of the V&VN and V&VN Department of Stoma care nurses.

The guideline will be introduced to non-members by means of regional ostomy networks and national symposia.

In addition the following groups will be informed of the existence of this guideline: manufacturers of ostomy products, medical specialist shops, Nefemed stoma materials interest group, FHI Medical specialist shop for Diabetes, Incontinence & Ostomy interest group (DISC), Dutch health insurance companies, the Ministry of Health, Welfare and Sport (VWS), the Central counselling organisation (for self-care), the V&VN, other professional associations with affinity for ostomy as well as academic journals.

8.3 Implementation and evaluation
Implementation
Implementation is described as 'a process-oriented and planned implementation or renewal and/or improvements (of proven value) with the aim that these become structurally integrated in (professional) actions, in the functioning of the organization(s) or in the structure of health care' (Hulscher, 2000 in Grol, 2007).

Grol (2007) describes different approaches to implementing improvements within self-care. A distinction is made between two approaches. An approach that focuses on internal processes (educational, epidemiological and marketing) and an approach that focuses on external factors

(such as external influence, social interaction, management and control and coercion).
Fleuren (2004) implores that the determinants (characteristics) that obstruct or accept the introduction of an implementation, in this case the guideline on ostomy, be defined. By means of literature review and delphi study, 49 determinants were identified. These were clustered based on characteristics of social/political context, organization, users and the characteristics of the specific innovation.

On the whole, Grol makes a distinction between two approaches of implementation: the rational model and the participation model.

Rational model	Participation model
• Implementation proceeds linearly	• Implementation proceeds gradually
• Clear starting point of implementation	• Unclear starting point
• Directed from the top-down	• Directed from practical experience level
• Driven by demand and technology	• Driven by need of technology
• Often positive towards technology	• Neutral to innovation
• No attention to diversity of the needs in practise	• No attention to macro processes, risk of implementation of suboptimal technology

Approaches to implementation (Van Woerkom, 1998 in Grol 2006)

Elements from both models were used for the development of this guideline. This is consistent with the advice of the Dutch Board of Health (2000, in Grol 2006) which states that "optimizing patient care is a two-way dialogue between science and practice".

By engaging with, and making use of, the target group problems with regard to implementation will most likely be reduced and the guideline will be accepted sooner. This will benefit the quality of patient care. This means that the professional group of (stoma care) nurses will oversee the systematic and process-based implementation of the guideline in their own institution. For this purpose protocols and work instructions (within the organization) will have to be adapted or developed in accordance to the guideline (recommendations).

To facilitate the implementation the recommendations have been compiled. In addition, some attachments from the guideline are available as a separate document to be used as a tool in daily practice.

Evaluation
The working group is of the opinion that the guideline should be evaluated regularly to keep up with scientific developments. The board of the V&VN Department of Stoma care nurses assigned the task of evaluation to its own technical committee. The working group is of the opinion that the guideline requires an update every five years in order to comply with the latest scientific developments. If important evidence arises within the period of five years, a decision could be made to move revision of the guideline forward.

The members of V&VN Department of Stoma care nurses are responsible for the evaluation of (implementation of) the guideline in their work setting. They can also report any amendments and additions via the website to the technical committee.

The guideline will be a recurring topic at the annual meeting of the V&VN Department of Stoma care nurses.

8.4 Assessment in practice

This guideline is intended to support stoma care provided by nurses and care providers. The scientific findings are translated into practice by means of recommendations. These recommendations should improve the quality of stoma care. To measure the quality of stoma care, indicators are used. Indicators are instruments that can be used to evaluate the effect of a recommendation.

By using indicators, it is possible to check whether the provided care meets the current requirements. The indicators are divided into structure, process and outcome of indicators. They are determined by a multidisciplinary working group and will be attached to the electronic version of this guideline before November 2013.

Chapter 9 Lacunae

While searching for answers to the starting point questions and the evidence, the working group encountered several lacunae or gaps in the available knowledge and evidence. More research is therefore to be conducted. The knowledge and evidence gaps are listed below and, if necessary, briefly explained.

The topics on which no or insufficient evidence has been found:
a. Incidence and prevalence.
b. Unambiguous description of complications and associated nursing interventions.
c. Comparison of different instruments for assessing peristomal problems.
d. Which stoma materials are suitable in which situations?
e. Which stoma aids are suitable for which problems or complications?
f. Criteria with regard to the number of stoma materials to be used.
g. Stoma irrigation.
h. What level of training is required for what type of stoma care?
i. How much staffing is required?

Explanation
• Incidence and prevalence (point a):
To obtain reliable incidence and prevalence figures, the subject of ostomy must be entered as a separate item in care registration systems.
• Description of complications and associated interventions, and the measuring instrument to be used (points b and c):
In some articles a start was made on formulating unequivocal definitions for complications and the appropriate sensible interventions for each. These can be used as basis for further development of the Dutch situation.
In this guideline a few measuring instruments were named. Some had been examined individually, however, a comparative study of multiple instruments was not found. The working group recommends research into, and assessment of, all existing instruments, both nationally and internationally, with the aim to improve the quality and reliability of classification of skin disorders.
A decision tree for parastomal hernia is utilized in the Netherlands. Currently, this instrument is the best available, but it is not evidence-based (PON, 2006). More research is required to substantiate interventions and prevention measures.
Insufficient evidence was found for the manner in which urine sampling for bacteriological examination from a urostomy should be done. This concerns a method where the results provide reliable information.
• Materials and use (point d, e and f):
There is a lack of objective information about the composition of the materials and subsequently knowledge of the properties, for example: moisture retaining capacity, wear time, etc.
In addition research is required to obtain evidence in establishing which stoma materials and stoma aids are needed for which problems or complications.

• No evidence was found with respect to the amount of water, frequency of rinsing, and duration of flushing in irrigating the stoma (point g):

Irrigation through a stoma is applied by many ostomates, however, no protocol or consensus on the methods was found.

• Education and availability of care providers in stoma care (points h and i):

Some studies were found with regard to the desired skills level within general nursing care, but studies conducted specifically within stoma care were not found.

Questions that can be asked here: what level of education is desirable in stoma care? What are the minimum requirements with regard to practical experience and theoretical level expected from the stoma care nurse and nurses and care providers working in stoma care?

Furthermore, there is a lack of evidence with regard to the availability of the required number of working-hours of a stoma care nurse in relation to the supply of stoma patients.

The working group recommends that the professional group should determine and come to an agreement on the minimum requirements for training, experience and on-going education of the various care providers. The profession should also decide on follow-up training en life-long professional education.

These different knowledge and evidence gaps require multiple forms of research. The working group recommends further research; the topic to be research should determine the appropriate research method.

Appendix I Members of working group and the sounding board group

The members of the working group are:

Mrs. H.G. (Giny) Baas
Nursing consultant stoma care, Martini Hospital Groningen

Mr. H.F. (Henk) Beekhuizen
Specialised nurse stoma care, wound management, continence and bladder function;
CombiCare Waddinxveen

Mrs. T. (Thea) Bremer - Goossens
Specialised nurse stoma care and continence; Evean

Mrs. J.E.C. (Conny) de Buck VS
Specialist nurse MDL; ZorgSaam Zeeland Flanders

Mrs. M. (Miranda) Broekhof
Specialised nurse stoma care, wound management, continence and bladder function; MediReva
Maastricht

Mrs. M.P. (Marianne) den Hertog
Nursing consultant stoma care; St. Antonius Hospital Nieuwegein

Mrs. M.A. (Rietje) Klievink VS
Specialist nurse oncology surgery; Riverenland Hospital Tiel.
Previously stoma care and wound management nurse; Diakonessenhuis Utrecht

Mrs. S.I. (Sigrun) Klok
Nursing consultant stoma care; Hospital Gelderse Vallei, Ede

Mrs. I.M. (Iris) Mast
Specialised nurse stoma care, wound management and pressure ulcers; Zaans Medical Centre
Zaandam

Mrs. J.H. (Ineke) Rook
Specialised nurse stoma care and wound management; Diaconessenhuis Leiden

Mrs. J.J.G. (Jolanda) Smelt MANP
Specialised nurse stoma care, wound management, continence and bladder function;
CombiCare, Waddinxveen

Counselling with respect to the methodology was offered by:

Mrs. G.J.J.W. (Gerrie) Bours
Nurse, nursing scientist and epidemiologist. Senior lecturer at Zuyd College, Faculty of Health and Care and senior researcher at the research group autonomy and participation in people with a chronic disease of the college. She lectures at the University of Maastricht, Department of Health Services Research/School of Public Health and Primary Care (Caphri).

Members of the sounding board group are:

Mrs. J.A. (Anne) Braakman
Director Dutch Ostomy Association (NSV)

Dr. W.M.U. (Helma) van Grevenstein
Gastrointestinal surgeon, UMC Utrecht, Dutch Association for Surgery (NVVH)

Prof. S. (Simon) Horenblas
Head of department of urology, Dutch Cancer Institute - Antoni van Leeuwenhoek Hospital Dutch Association for Urology (NCE)

Dr. R. (Ronald) Houwing
Dermatologist, Deventer Hospital, Dutch Society of Dermatology and Venereology (in adds)

Mrs. C.M.M. (Pien) Lelie
Dietician, Hospital Gelderse Vallei, Ede, Dutch Association of Dieticians (NVD)

Mr. M.R. (Maarten) Tempelaar
Board member Dutch Ostomy Association (NSV)

Dr. M.A.M.T. (Marc) Verhagen
Gastroenterologist, Diakonessenhuis Utrecht, Dutch Association of Gastroenterologists (NVMDL)

All delegated by their (professional) association.

Member of the sounding board group on personal title:
Mrs. H. (Hanny) Cobussen- Boekhorst MANP
Specialist nurse continence and urostomy care in the Department of Urology, UMC St. Radboud, Nijmegen. Involved in development of several evidence-based guidelines and the European Association of Urology Nurses (EAUN)

Appendix II Levels of Evidence;

Classification of methodological quality and individual studies

	Intervention	Diagnostic accuracy study	Damage or side effects, etiology, prognosis *
A1	Systematic review of at least two independently conducted A2 level studies		
A2	High standard, sufficiently sized, randomized, double-blind, comparative, clinical studies	Study relative to a referenced test ('golden standard') with predefined cut-off values and independent assessment of the results of test and golden standard, on a sufficiently large series of consecutive patients, all of them having had the index and reference test	Prospective cohort study of sufficient size and follow-up, where 'confounding' was adequately controlled and selective follow-up was sufficiently excluded.
B	Comparative study, but not including all the features listed under A2 (this includes patient-control studies, cohort studies)	Study relative to a referenced test, but not with all the features listed under A2	Prospective cohort study, but not including all the features listed under A2 or retrospective cohort or patient-control study
C	Non-comparative study		
D	Expert opinion		

*This classification only applies to situations where controlled trials are not possible due to ethical or other reasons. If they are possible, the classification applies to interventions.

Level of Conclusion

	Conclusion based on
1	Study of level A1 or at least two independently conducted studies of level A2
2	One study of level A2 or at least two independently conducted studies of level B
3	One study of level B or C
4	Expert opinion

Appendix III Search terms

adhesive
adult Ostomy Patient
advanced practice nurse
allergic
allergy
appliance
care nurse
classifying complications
clinical nurse
clinical nurse specialist
community care
community nurse
complications
continuing
continuing care
continuing nursing
continuity
continuity care
continuity of care
convex
coping
definition
dehydration
dermatitis
discharge
district nurse
eczema
education
educational level
erosion
fistula
flatus
flux
follow-up
frequency complications
granuloma
hernia
herniation ostomy
high output
hospital
hospital discharge

hyperkeratosis
hyperpigmentation
information
localization
maceration
necrosis
nurse
nurse practitioner
nurse specialist
nursing care
nursing specialist
nursing student
obstipation
occlusion
oedema
ostomy
ostomy bag
ostomy care
ostomy management
ostomy necrosis
ostomy nurse
ostomy nurse preventive
ostomy nursing care
ostomy retraction
ostomy siting
outpatient care
parastomal hernia
parastomal hernia definition
patient education
peristomal skin condition
peristomal skin disorders
postoperative ostomy care standard
postoperative phase
postoperative
post surgery
pouch
pouch system
practice nurse
pregnancy
preoperative
preparation

presurgery
preventing and treating parastomal hernia
prolaps
pyoderma
registered nurse
rehabilitation
retracted stoma
retraction
RN
school nurse
separation
siting
skin
skin excoriation
skin stripping
skin damage
skin irritation
specialist nurse
stenosis

stoma
stoma bag
stoma care
stoma care nursing
stoma management
stoma management skills
stoma mucocutaneous separation
stoma nurse
stoma prolapse
stoma siting
stoma care nursing
stomal complications definitions
stoma necrosis
student nurse
teaching
ulcus
wound, ostomy, and continence nurse
wound, ostomy, and continence specialist nurse

Appendix IV List of definitions and abbreviations

• **Adequate**
Suitable for the intended purpose;
• **Adults:**
Age 18 years older;
• **Body image**
Body image: the overall concept, including conscious and unconscious feelings, thoughts and perceptions, that a person has his or her own body as an object in space independent and distinctive from other objects (www.encyclo.co.uk/search. ipp dated 4-7-12);
• **Candidiasis**
An overgrowth of fungal organisms (Candida) sufficient to cause infection of the skin around the stoma;
• **Care pathway**
Collection of methods and tools to align the processes of care for a specific group of patients performed by outpatient or clinical multi- and inter-disciplinary teams (translation of www.encyclo.nl/begrip/zorgpaden dd.p 4-7-12);
• **Case manager**
 A nurse, doctor or social worker who works with patients, providers and insurers to co-ordinate all services deemed necessary to provide the patient with a plan of medical necessary and appropriate health care;
• **Colorectal**
With regard to the large intestine (colon) and rectum;
• **Colostomy**
Colo refers to the location of the stoma in the colon (large intestine), The ideal end stoma has a round shape, red colouring, similar to oral mucosa and protrudes 1 to 1.5 inches above skin level;
• **Contact dermatitis**
Damage to the skin by exposure to faeces, urine or chemical preparations;
• **Continent stoma**
A stoma for urine or loose stools as an outlet of an internal artificial reservoir of the small intestine, which is to be emptied with the aid of a catheter. This stoma is not covered by this guideline;
• **Convex/convexity**
Descending bowl-shaped surface of the skin barrier causing increased pressure on the peristomal skin directly to the stoma;
• **Coping**
The way someone deals with problems and events, as well as dealing with intense thoughts or feelings (translation of www.encyclo.nl/zoek.php?woord = coping dated 4-7-12.);
• **Counselling**
Giving information through communication, allowing an interested person to come to a well-balanced decision and forming opinions in a concrete situation;
• **Discharge phase**
Phase of preparing the patient for discharge from hospital;
• **Education**
The conscious and deliberate creation of conditions and organization of activities and learning for some time, to increase knowledge and insight (www.mijnwoordenboek.nl/translation/EN/EN/education dd 10-11. - 11);
• **End stoma**
The proximal cut end of the colon is advanced and sutured to the abdominal wall to form a stoma (Kuipers, NTVG 2001);

- **Evidence-based**
Based on data from quantitative and/or qualitative scientific research (translation of www.encyclo.nl/zoek.php?woord=evidence+ dated 4-7-12.);
- **Fascia opening**
Opening in the muscle layer of the abdominal wall where the stoma is advanced to the outside;
- **Fistula**
Abnormal communication between the stoma and the surrounding tissue or in the stoma other than the lumen;
- **Folliculitis**
Inflammation of hair follicles on the peristomal skin;
- **Follow-up**
Regular follow-up of patients (translation of www.encyclo.nl/zoek.php woord = follow-up dated 4-7-12.);
- **FTE**
Full-time equivalent. Unit indicating work load or staff employment. (translation of Http://nl.wikipedia.org/wiki/Fte. Dated 25-7-2012.);
- **Granuloma**
Excessive tissue occurring at the skin/stoma base in areas of retained or reactive suture material;
- **High-output**
High production of a bowel stoma of more than 1 litre per 24 hours;
- **Incidence**
The number of new cases of a disease, or the number of people that develop a certain disease for the first time, during a specific period of time;
- **Indicator**
Evidences that might lead to certain conclusions. More specific term: performance indicators (translation of indicators www.encyclo.nl/zoek.php?woord = dd 4-7-12.);
- **Ileostomy**
Ileo refers to the location of the stoma in the ileum (small intestine);
- **Implementation**
Various activities and measures necessary to introduce and take into use the guideline (translation of www.woorden-boek.nl/woord/implementation dated 4-7-12.);
- **Information**
Data that increases knowledge. (translation of www.woorden.org/word/information dated 10-11-11.);
- **Intervention**
A set of activities that aid workers utilize for and with clients (groups) to prevent or solve problems in order to help promote and maintain health and well-being (translation of www.encyclo.nl/zoek.php?woord=interventie dd. 4 -7-12);
- **Integrated care**
Care where the different parties are aligned resulting in a coherent supply, focusing on the needs of each patient
(translation of www.encyclo.nl/zoek.php?woord = integrated care dd 4-7-12.);
- **Irrigation**
Flushing of the colon on a regular basis with water and help of special materials, so that the stoma is free from effluent for 24 up to 48 hours;
- **Leakage**
Stool or urine that penetrates between the skin barrier and the skin, as a result of a complication or other problem;
- **Loop stoma**
Stoma that is constructed by taking a bowel loop through an opening in the abdominal wall, open it, and attach it to the skin on the outside. This results in two openings next to each other, one for discharge of stool and the other for mucous (Kuipers, NTVG 2001);
- **(Mucocutaneaus) separation**
Detachment of stomal tissue from the surrounding peristomal skin;

• Mucus Fistula
A mucus fistula is always the second stoma to be constructed, offers the opportunity to   drain bowel mucus and waste from the disabled part of the bowel since it can no longer be excreted through the anus (Burch, 2008);

• Musculus rectus abdominus
Straight abdominal muscle that runs from the chest to the pubic bone and in which an opening is made during surgery to advance the stoma;

• Necrosis
Death of the stomal tissue resulting from impaired blood flow;

• Obesity
Severe obesity is a chronic disease in which the body stores so much fat that it can cause physical problems. A person with a Body Mass Index (BMI) > 30iis considered to be obese (translation of www.encie.nl/definition/Obesity dated 4-7-2012.);

• Obstruction
Blockage of the stomal passage resulting in no stool and/or flatus;

• Oedema
Accumulation of fluid in the stoma causing the stoma to enlarge;

• Opinion piece
 Publication in which the opinion of the author is expressed;

• Obstipation
 Accumulation of faeces in the colon, resulting in a delayed excretion of hard, dry stools through the stoma;

• Output
 The stoma production, also called effluent;

• Pancaking
 Faeces does not move down into the stoma bag, but remains around the stoma;

• Parastomal hernia
 Defect in the abdominal fascia that allows the intestine to bulge into the parastomal area;

• Perineum wound
 Wound after rectum amputation in the anal cleft. The perineum is the area between the anus and the scrotum in the male and the anus and vulva in the female (translation of http://nl.wikipedia.org/wiki/perineum dated 4-7-12);

• Peristomal skin
 Skin around the stoma underneath the skin barrier;

• Permanent stoma
 A stoma where the medical intervention has been such, that due to technical or medical reasons, the natural opening cannot be restored;

• Physical wholeness
A person experiences his body as whole, if he can be the body that he has (translation of http://www.nwo.nl/nwohome.nsf/pages/NWOP_8JGJZ9 dated 11-3-2012.);

• PLISSIT
A conversation model, the letters form an anagram for Permission, Low threshold Information, Specific Suggestions, Intensive Therapy;

• Postoperative clinical phase
The period from the surgery until discharge from hospital, this phase overlaps into the discharge phase;

• Pouch
An artificially created reservoir for collecting stool, connected to the anus. A pouch is not covered by this guideline;

• Preoperative phase
The phase prior to surgery in which a stoma is likely to be constructed;

- **Prevalence**
The total number of people with an illness, disability or condition present in the population at a given time. (translation of Http://www.encyclo en, June 2011.);
- **Prolapse**
A telescoping of the intestine through the stoma;
- **Pseudo verrucous lesions**
Wart-like lesions in the peristomal area caused by chronic moisture exposure and irritation;
- **Pyoderma gangrenosum**
An ulcerative skin condition of unknown etiology occurring around the stoma;
- **Retraction**
The disappearance of normal stomal protrusion in line with or below skin level;
- **Self-care**
Self-care is a term taken from nursing indicating the extent to which a patient (or person in need of care) can take care of himself. Self-care is described as "all the care that a person spends on upgrading and meeting his own needs". In ostomy it refers to the extent to which the ostomate is able to manage his stoma (translation of www.encyclo.nl/begrip/zelfzorg dd 4-7-12.);
- **Self-efficacy**
Belief in the own abilities, self-confidence;
- **Skin barrier**
The adhesive part of the stoma appliance;
- **Splints**
Thin tubes in the upper urinary tract to protect the anastomoses between the ureters and the bowel during the postoperative period;
- **Stenosis**
Impairment of effluent drainage due to narrowing or contraction of the stomal tissue at the level of the skin or fascia;
- **Stoma**
 Unnatural and/or artificial opening which connects a body cavity to the outside world;
- **Stoma accessories**
All other materials (except stoma appliances) which may be necessary to take care of the stoma;
- **Stoma appliance**
Skin barrier and stoma bag;
- **Stoma bag**
Part of the stoma appliance that collects the output;
- **Stoma care nurse**
 Nurse who is specialised in stoma care;
- **Stomal siting**
The choice of the ideal location for an abdominal stoma prior to surgery to prevent stoma complications and problems with adhesion of the stoma material;
- **Stomal trauma**
Laceration of stomal mucosa, usually by pressure or physical force;
- **Stomal varices** (Caput medusae)
Large portosystemic venous collateral blood vessels that are visible next to the stoma;
- **Temporary stoma**
Stoma that is constructed with the intention to be removed again at a later stage (NTVG Kuijpers, 2001);
- **Training**
Learning, improving or changing social, cognitive and psycho-motor skills (www.mijnwoordenboek.nl/translation/EN/EN/training) dd. 10-11-11);
- **Transverse colon**
Horizontal part of the large intestine (colon);

• Urostomy

In a urostomy, the two ureters are transplanted into an isolated piece of ileum (operation according to Bricker). One end is closed and the other end of the bowel section is attached as a stoma into the abdominal wall;

• Validate

Establish that the equipment/method is suitable for the purpose. Also, the process in order to achieve an acceptable quality of a given fact (translation of www.encyclo.nl/zoek.php?woord = valideren dd 4-7-12.);

List of abbreviations

ADL	General Daily Living;
AGREE	Appraisal of Guidelines for Research and Evaluation, a tool for assessing guidelines;
ASCRS	American Society of Colon & Rectal Surgeons;
CBO	Centraal BegeleidingsOrgaan;
DBC	The complete trajectory from diagnosis to treatment
DET score	Discolouring Erosion Tissue overgrowth. A measuring instrument for peristomal skin conditions.
DICA	Dutch Institute for Clinical Auditing;
DOT	DBC Towards Transparency. Expenses claims for care products. A diagnosis treatment combination;
DSCA	Dutch Surgical Colorectal Audit
EAUN	European Association of Urology Nurses;
EBRO	Evidence-based guideline development;
EPD	Electronic patient file;
FAP	Familial adenomatous polyposis;
ICF	International Classification of Functioning, Disability and Health;
MANP	Master advanced Nursing Practice (nurse specialist);
NSV	Nederlandse Stomavereniging (Dutch Ostomy Association);
ORS	Oral Rehydration Salts;
RNAO	Registered Nurses Association of Ontario (Canada);
RIVM	National Institute for Public Health and Environment;
SACS instrument	Anagram for: Studio Alterazioni cutanée Stomali. A measuring instrument designed for a study on peristomal skin lesions in Italy;
VIKC	Association of Comprehensive Cancer Centres, the national association of the eight comprehensive cancer centres in the Netherlands;
V&VN	Association of nurses and care providers Netherlands, an umbrella organization.
V&VN stoma care nurses	Part of the V&VN, professional association for stoma nurses
WOCN	Wound Ostomy Continence Nurses Society (United States of America).

Appendix V Indications

There are many different reasons why a stoma becomes necessary. The various types of stomata all have different indications (in alphabetical order).

Indications for the construction of a permanent or temporary colostomy are:
• Protection anastomosis;
• Colitis ulcerosa;
• Congenital abnormalities;
• Enterocutaneous fistulas;
• Iatrogenic (due to complications after surgery);
• Incontinence;
• Ischemic bowel;
• Neurological disorders (multiple sclerosis, spinal cord injury);
• Obstipation;
• Obstruction;
• Inflammation/(perforated) diverticulitis;
• Perianal problems;
• Trauma;
• Tumors;
• Crohn's disease.

Indications for the construction of a permanent or temporary ileostomy are:
• Protection anastomosis;
• Colitis ulcerosa;
• Enterocutaneous fistulas;
• Familial adenomatous polyposis (ΓAP),
• Iatrogenic (due to complications after surgery)
• Necrosis;
• Neurological disorders (multiple sclerosis, spinal cord injury);
• Inflammation/(perforated) diverticulitis;
• Perianal problems;
• Slow transit issues;
• Trauma;
• Tumors;
• Crohn's disease.

Indications for the construction of a urostomy are:
• Congenital abnormalities;
• Fistula (colovesical or vesicocutaneous);
• Iatrogenic (due to complications after surgery);
• Incontinence;
• Interstitial Cystitis;
• Neurological disorders (Multiple sclerosis, spinal cord injury);
• Shrunken bladder;
• Trauma;
• Tumors.

Appendix VI Preoperative counselling and information topics

Evaluate the consultation between patient and doctor, what does the patient know about his illness and the surgery?
• Diagnosis, explanation of disease, genetics
• Essential issues related to the planned surgery, surgical technique
• Possible complications of surgery
• Expected duration of hospital stay
• Bowel preparation

What is a stoma?
• Explain anatomy and physiology
• Siting of the stoma/positioning
• Appearance of the stoma
• Experiencing the stoma
• Characteristics of the stoma and the output

Information about stoma material
• Explain different types of stoma appliances and accessories

• Reimbursement
• Practicing with stoma appliances

Self-care/management
• Learning the self-care
• Peristomal skin care, hair removal
• Odour/gas forming
• Involving the spouse and/or relatives

Consequences of having a stoma
• Rectal loss of mucus and faeces
• Possible (early and late) complications of a stoma
• Phantom feeling

Discharge/aftercare
• Ordering/delivery of stoma materials
• Task stoma nurse/community nurse
• Explanation about accessibility of the outpatient clinic and what the patient can expect from the stoma nurse

Consequences for everyday life
• Nutrition, diet
• Social aspects
• Psychological aspects
• Changed self-image
• Showering, bathing and swimming
• Clothing
• Work
• Sports/hobbies
• Holidays
• Sexuality/intimacy
• Pregnancy, fertility

- Medication
- Irrigation
- Abdominal exercises
- Home situation

Educational materials include:
- Folder with drawings of anatomy
- Photographs of various stomata
- Books
- Internet
- CD-ROMs, film
- Brochures
- The Dutch Ostomy Association

Appendix VII Working method to determine the site of the stoma

Action	Explanation
Gather relevant information about the condition and the surgery	Different stomata require different sitings
Gather specific information on the patient: Lifestyle, occupation, body shape, religion, orthopaedic aids, hobbies and sports	If using an aid i.e. wheelchair or orthopaedic aid, the site marking should be carried out while the patient is sitting in the wheelchair or using the aid. The wheelchair or aid may not hinder adequate collecting of the effluent
Inform the patient about the purpose and method of the operation and make a joined decision on the siting of the stoma	Consent promotes acceptance
Let the patient lie down and hitch up the abdomen	Stomas will be placed within the rectus abdominus
Make an imaginary triangle between the umbilicus, pelvic crest and os pubis; for a place on the transverse colon: make an imaginary triangle between the umbilicus, pelvic crest and rib cage. Mark the place as an orientation point marking where the stoma might possibly come out	The stoma will preferably be constructed within this triangle, leaving sufficient space for the skin barrier
Let the patient bend over and sit down, to register any skin folds or dents	For adequately applying the stoma material and to prevent leakage caused by skin folds and dents
Discuss clothing habits in relation to the stoma site	Prevent disappointment and limitation of daily life and habits as well as complications
Check if the site is visible and accessible to the patient in different positions	The patient can take care of his stoma
Place a sample bag over the orientation marking and evaluate this with the patient	See how the appliance reacts to movement and what the relation is to scars, navel, incision line and the structure of the skeleton
Discuss the chosen site with the patient	The patient agrees to the site and understands the choice
Do the final marking	Ensure that the surgeon clearly sees the marked site, *also after disinfection*
Do not use tattoo ink	Tattoo ink is a permanent marking
Inform the surgeon if the site is different to what would be expected	This to prevent the surgeon from using the usual site

Appendix VIII Postoperative stoma checklist

• Vitality: Colour of the stoma and aspect of mucosa, oedema
• Stoma height and size
• Location
• Whether or not a bridge is present
• Sutures
• Splints present in urostomy and production
• Check stoma appliance
• Condition of peristomal skin
• Functioning of intestines or kidneys: excretion of the stoma (quantity, consistency, flatus)

Observation	Normal aspect/normal values
Vitality	Colour of mucosa: pink to bright red
	Aspect mucosa: moist
	Oedema: presence of oedema is normal
Stoma height and size	Gradual decrease is normal
Location	On the marked site
Bridge	Present or not
Sutures	Are functional
Check stoma appliance	Functional, properly applied and suitable for the effluent
Condition of the peristomal skin	Slight redness under the entire skin barrier is normal after removing the skin barrier, this fades within 5 minutes

Discharge from the stoma

Type of stoma	Type of observation	Normal values
Colostomy	Start	After 1-4 days, depending on bowel preparation, peristalsis, medication
	Quantity	100-500 grams per 24 hours depending on the location on the colon
	Colour	Light brown to dark brown
	Consistency	Gruel to firm stool
	Other	Flatus is normal
Ileostomy	Start	Within 24 hours, guided by clinical impression
	Quantity	750-1000 ml per 24 hours
	Colour	Dark yellow to green and brown
	Consistency	Watery to gruel-like, sometimes foamy
	Other	Flatus is normal
Urostomy	Start	Immediately postoperatively, every splint has to produce
	Quantity	Minimal 30 ml per hour
	Colour	Bright straw yellow in colour and almost odourless
	Consistency	Flakes could be present
	Other	Splints are present, one splint per kidney

Appendix IX Roadmap for self-care education

Preoperative phase

The patient has:		Initial
1	Received instruction on the method of stoma care	
2	Seen and handled the stoma appliances	
3	Was offered the possibility to wear and practice with the appliance	

Introduction to the stoma

The patient has:		Initial
1	Participated in stoma care by observing	
2	Touched the stoma with gauze	
3	Received instruction on the method of stoma care	
4	Observed the emptying of the bag	

Instruction Phase

The patient knows:		Initial
1	When the stoma appliance should be emptied or changed	
2	Which materials should be at hand when managing the stoma	
3	How to empty the stoma appliance	

The patient:		Initial
1	Empties the stoma appliance under supervision	
2	Removes the stoma appliance under supervision	
3	Cleans the stoma and peristomal skin under supervision	
4	Checks and measures the opening that has to be cut in the skin barrier under supervision	
5	Cuts the appropriate opening in the skin barrier under supervision	
6	Applies the stoma appliance under supervision	
7	In the case of a two-piece system, changes the bag under supervision	

The patient knows:		Initial
1	How to clean and dry the peristomal skin	
2	What normal peristomal skin looks like	
3	How to take care of the peristomal skin	
4	How to dispose of collecting material	
5	In a urostomy, how to independently apply a night drainage bag, remove and clean it	

The patient:		Initial
1	Independently empties the stoma bag	
2	Independently removes the stoma appliance	
3	Independently cleans the stoma and the peristomal skin	
4	Independently checks and measures the opening to be cut in the skin barrier	
5	Independently cuts the appropriate opening in the skin barrier	
6	Independently applies the stoma appliance	
7	In case of a two-piece system, independently changes the stoma bag	

Appendix X Decision tree for choice of stoma materials

Patient information:

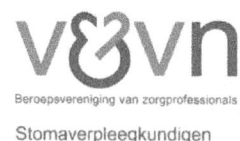

Date :....-....-....

Stoma Care Nurse: ....

1.Indication	
Description of problem	
2. Characterisation	
A. Patient characteristics	
A1. Physical functioning	
A2. Activities	
A3. Physical characteristics	
A4. Situation at home	
A5. Current illnesses and treatments	
A6.Medication	
B. Personal preference	
C. Stoma features	
C1. Colour/blood supply of stoma	
C2. Shape/size of stoma	
C3. Height of stoma	
C4. Location of stoma	
C5. Condition of peristomal skin	
C6. Output of stoma	

D. Product requirements	
System: ☐ 1-piece ☐ 2-piece **Skin barrier:** ☐ plane barrier ☐ convex ☐ stationary flange ☐ floating ☐ pre-formed ☐ fit to cut ☐ mouldable ☐ thickened skin ☐ adhesive closure ☐ ring closure **Collecting bags:** ☐ transparent ☐ opaque ☐ filter ☐ no filter ☐ flushable	**Fastening:** ☐ closed ☐ integrated closure ☐ clip ☐ tap **Volume of bag:** Colo/uro: ☐ to 300ml ☐ 300-600ml ☐ > 600ml Ileo: ☐ to 400ml ☐ 400-700ml ☐ > 700ml **Accessories:** ☐ skin protection ☐ fillers ☐ thickening agents ☐ fixtures ☐ odour neutralizers ☐ other ....
3. Selecting	
Choice of brand and type	
4. Order	
Material and order instruction	Supplier: ....
5. Evaluation	Evaluation date: ....-....-.... Findings: .... Goal achieved ☐ yes ☐ if no, adjust!

Explanation:

1. **Indication: Type of stoma:** colo- ileo- or urostomy
   Describing the problem: first choice of material, leakage, etc.

2. **A1. Physical functioning**: limitations that can influence stoma management: vision, dexterity, wheelchair bound, bedridden, etc.
   A3. Physical characteristics: characteristics of the skin such as sensitivity, prone to allergies, moisture, patient's build etc.
   A4. Situation at home: spouse: yes/no, care given by relatives etc.
   A5. Illnesses: also psychological disorders, dementia and fear, diabetes, Parkinson's.
   C5. Condition of peristomal skin: redness, stripped skin, scars, skin folds, etc.
   D. Product Requirements: Conclusion of the characterisation; in other words the material requirements that should be met. (Tick off choice)

5. **Evaluation**: in case of problems.

Appendix XI   Hospital discharge checklist

The stoma care nurse:

	Action	Initial	Date
1.	Checks the stoma, peristomal skin and stoma production Checks the choice of materials Hands the patient an appropriate template		
2.	Provides information and education materials specially aimed at the ostomate * General stoma instruction * Information on patient associations * Checks if the patient understands the do's & don'ts * Nutritional advice		
3.	Checks if (community) care is organised after discharge		
4.	Transferal to community care/institution: see Appendix XIV		
5.	Arranges the supply of stoma materials * Supplier is known, materials are ordered *Patient knows contact details of suppliers and how to order. * Accountability for reimbursement of the materials from the insurance		
6.	Supplies the ostomate with sufficient stoma materials to last until the first delivery		
7.	Makes sure that the outpatient consultation with the stoma care nurse is planned * Supplies the ostomate with phone numbers and information on where the nurse can be reached * Explains in which situations the stoma care nurse can be consulted * Explains what the ostomate should do in acute situations, who can be called * Explains about the follow-up		

Appendix XII Specific nutritional aspects

Foods that form a risk for obstruction and obstipation when not chewed properly
• Coarse wheat bran, popcorn, seeds and nuts
• stringy meat or skin of sausage,
• Asparagus, mushrooms, chinese vegetables/over-cooked cabbage, corn cobs, celery, taugé, sauerkraut, pieces of pineapple, orange and dried fruit or fruit seeds.

Foods that can thicken the stool (in ileostomy with excessive production)
• Dry non-greasy starch and fibre products: such as bread, crackers
• Rice, pasta, potatoes.

Foods that increase the tempo of passage through the bowel
• Products rich in sugar and sugar substitutes (especially sorbitol or xylitol)
• Large amounts of fluids at one time or abundant fluid intake during a meal
• Coffee
• Onions, garlic and peppers
• Too much indigestible fibre, particularly uncooked vegetables, unpeeled fruit and vegetable and/or fruit juices

Additional advice in case of high-output
• 3 meals and 3 in-between meals with products that thicken the stool.
• Not more than 2.5 litres of fluids per 24 hour. Part of which consists of 1-3 sachets of ORS (oral rehydration salts). Optionally, when high-output lasts for a longer period of time, fluid intake should be limited, but in combination with infusion.
• Limit watery drinks and vary in types of beverages: up to 500cc milk drinks, up to 2 glasses (carbonated) lemonade and up to 2 glasses of fruit juice
• Increase salt intake

Foods rich in salt
• Salt
• Sprinkle aroma, soy sauce, soup, tomato ketchup, curry
• Soup, broth, vegetable and tomato juice
• Meat, (spreadable) cheese, salted fish
• ORS and a number of types of sports drink

Foods which can increase gas forming
• Legumes, onion, garlic, pepper, over-cooked cabbage
• Carbonated drinks, beer.
• Eggs.
• Chewing gum

Nutrition advice with an acidifying effect on urine production
• Products that contain a lot of animal protein, besides meat also cheese
• Lentils and legumes
• Limit the use of citrus fruits and juices

Foods that could cause discoloration or different odour of the effluent
• Garlic, asparagus, beetroot, spinach, leeks and over cooked cabbage
• Fish and eggs, cheese
• Vitamin B tablets, iron preparations

Sources:	
Author title	level
Fulham, J. (2008).Providing dietary advice for the individual with a stoma. *British journal of nursing, 17(2), 22-27.*	D
Burch, J. (2005). The pre- and postoperative nursing care for patients with a stoma. *British journal of nursing, 14(6), 310-318.*	D
Sica, J. & Burch, J. (2007). Management of bowel failure and high-output stomas. *British journal of nursing, 16(13), 772- 777.*	D
Burch, J. (2005). Stoma complications encountered in the community, AZ. *British Journal of community nursing, 10(7), 324-329.*	D
Burch, J. (2007). Obstipation and flatulence management for stoma patients. *British journal of community nursing, 12(10), 449-452.*	D
Burch, J. (2006). Nutrition and the ostomate: input, output and absorption. *British journal of community nursing, 11(8), 349-351.*	D
Doughty, D. (2005). Principles of ostomy management in oncology patients. *The journal of supportive oncology, 3(1), 59-69.*	D
Burch, J. (2008). Nutrition for people with stomas. 2: An overview of dietary advice. *Nursing times, 104(49), 26-27.* www.nursingtimes.net	D
Welink- Lamberts B., Werkgroep CHIODAZ (2007). Nieuwe dieetbehandelingsrichtlijn ileostomy. *Ned. tijdschrift voor voeding & diëtiek 62(3), 7-10*	D
Geng, V., Cobussen, H., Fillingham, S., Holroyd, S., Kiesbye, B., Vahr, S. (2009). Good practice in health care: incontinent urstomy. *European association of urology nurses.* EAUN. http://www.uoweb.org/professional-resources/guidelines/	AGREE
Registered nurses' association of Ontario. RNAO (2009) Ostomy care and management. Clinical best practice guidelines. *http://rnao.ca/sites/rnao-ca/files/Stoma care_Care__Management.pdf*	

Appendix XIII   Complications and other problems

In this Appendix various complications are discussed in more detail based on information from the publications used. The numbers in brackets refer to the articles from which the data is taken (see reference list at the end of this Appendix).
The following subjects are being discussed:
• Stomal problems: parastomal hernia, stoma prolaps, stoma necrosis, stoma separation, stoma retraction, stoma stenosis, stoma trauma, stoma fistula
• Peristomal problems: contact dermatitis, granuloma, candidiasis, folliculitis, pseudo verrucous lesions, pyoderma gangrenosum, stomal varices (caput medusae)
• Other problems with the stoma: leakage, pancaking, oedema
• Complications related to stool pattern: high output in bowel stoma, obstruction, obstipation, excessive gas forming

STOMAL PROBLEMS

Para(peri)stomal Hernia:
Definition
A defect of the abdominal fascia causing the intestine to protrude next to the stoma (8)
Incidence
0-66% (11, 20, 23, 30, 31)
Characteristics
• Swelling around the stoma which decreases in supine position and increases in sitting or standing position (2, 3)
• Causes discomfort and/or bloated feeling (2, 3, 27), painful stoma (31)
• Larger size of the stoma, and reduction of the stoma height (20, 31).
• Coughing or straining while performing an internal examination will reveal a fascia defect (2).
Cause and Risk Factors
• Inevitable consequence of the stoma construction (31)
• Increased risk by: age 70 years or above (23, 31), obesity (2, 11, 23, 31), diabetes (31) colostomy (16, 31)
• Causes: the abdominal wall is loaded too soon and too heavily particularly during the first two months after surgery, abnormalities of the abdominal wall (2), and/or chronic increased intra-abdominal pressure (31), stoma constructed in too large a fascia opening (2). The expert opinion is to construct the stoma in the rectus muscle (2), however, there is no significant evidence for this (16)
Consequences
• Leakage and skin disorders (2, 3, 38)
• Stoma care becomes more complicated (13)
• Bowel obstruction, bowel blockage (2)
• Risk of perforation in bowel irrigation (2.16)
• Reduced quality of life (20)
Nursing intervention and treatment
• Indication by stoma care nurse for referral to physician who makes a diagnoses (37).
• Refer short-term to the physician in signs of obstipation, bowel obstruction, perforation or unmanageable stoma (2) or severe psychological consequences.
• Conservative

Stoma prolaps
Definition
Telescoping of the intestine through the stoma (8)
Incidence
0-25% (14, 23, 30, 39)

Characteristics
Increased circumference and protrusion varying in length (2, 7)
Cause and Risk Factors
• Too large opening and insufficient attachment of the bowel to the abdominal wall, increased abdominal pressure (2, 7), obesity, abnormalities of the abdominal wall: underdeveloped and/or absence of abdominal muscles and fascia (2).
• Loop stoma on transverse colon (2, 7), in particular the distal bowel section (2)
Consequences
• Oedema (2, 7)
• Possible consequences: trauma, bleeding, ulceration of the mucus membrane (2, 7), ischemia (2, 7) necrosis (2) obstipation (2, 7), leakage and skin disorders (27, 38)
Nursing intervention and treatment
• Check the colour of the prolapse and the mucosa for damage and irritation (7)
• Try to decrease the oedema, apply cold compress (2, 3, 7, 8), and powdered sugar or (2, 7, 8)
• Manually reducing the stoma, and then support the abdominal wall with a stoma support belt (2, 7)
• Adjust stoma collecting material: flexible and flat material (2, 3)
• Refer to the surgeon in signs of ischemia, obstruction and inability to reduce the stoma (7)

Stoma necrosis
Definition
Death of stoma tissue due to impaired blood flow.
Incidence
0.4 to 12%, mainly as a complication immediately postoperatively (14, 23, 30, 39)
Characteristics
• The necrosis can be limited to a quadrant of the stoma or extends below the level of the fascia and affect stomal mucosa. (2, 8)
• Occurs usually within 24 hours after stoma construction (2, 7)
• A dark coloured stoma, purple-blue, brown to black, which
usually feels soft and flaccid (2, 7)
• Necrotic smell (2)
Cause and Risk Factors
• Too tight suturing of the stoma, insufficient mobilization of mesentery, embolism, oedema and/or postoperative abdominal distension (2, 7)
• Too thick abdominal wall (2)
• Too small opening in the skin barrier in postoperative oedema of the stoma (2, 7).
Consequences
• Loss of necrotic tissue (7)
• Mucocutaneous separation (2)
• Perforation and peritonitis (2)
• Scars and stenosis (2, 7)
Nursing intervention and treatment
• Alert or inform the physician (2, 7) in deeper necrosis (ischemic damage more than 2 cm deep) or extension of necrotic area (7)
• Investigation of the nature and severity of the necrosis by passing a small glass tube into the stoma and inspect mucosa with a penlight (2, 7)
• Regular monitoring for possible expansion is necessary (2, 7)
• Conservative treatment policy in limited necrosis above the fascial level (7)
• If necessary, removal of the necrotic tissue (8)

Stoma mucocutaneous separation
Definition
Detachment of stomal tissue from the surrounding peristomal skin (8)

Incidence
4-24% as an early complication (2, 14, 30, 38).
Characteristics
• Partial or circumferential separation of stoma mucosa and skin (2)
• Pain, burning sensation (2)
• Varies in depth and size (2)
Cause and Risk Factors
• Stoma was constructed under tension (2, 7, 38)
• Impaired wound healing and infection on the surface,
• Stomal necrosis (2, 7, 38).
• Use of convex system (2, 7)
Consequences
• Fistulas, common in ileostomata (7)
• Stenosis
Nursing intervention and treatment
• Flushing the wound area (7).
• Determination of the depth and extent (partially or circumferential) of the wound area and assess the tissue type at the base of the seperation (2, 7)
• Check for any fistulas (2, 7, 38)
• Choose wound healing products depending on the phase of the wound healing process (7, 38)
• Preferably use flat stoma material over the wound area and adjoining to the stoma (2, 7, 38). Depending on depth and amount of exudate the stoma opening can be kept open.

Stoma retraction
Definition
Disappearance of normal stoma protrusion in line with or below skin level (2, 8).
Incidence
• 4.5% - 40% as an early complication (2, 14, 30, 39)
• 1-24% as a late complication (2, 30)
Characteristics
• Retracted stoma. Retraction may increase when patient is sitting or lying (2, 7)
• The stoma appears like a concave defection on the abdomen, with creasing in the perostomal skin (2, 7)
• Stoma material does not adhere to the skin around the stoma properly ,because it does not touch the skin (13)
Cause and Risk Factors
• The stoma is constructed under tension, (2, 7, 33) increased BMI (> 30) (1)
• Impaired healing due to by postoperative swollen abdomen
• Premature removal of stoma bridge (2, 27, 33)
• Mucocutaneous separation and stoma necrosis (2, 7)
• Increase in body weight (27, 29)
Possible Consequences
Shortened wear time of the material, leakage (3, 7)
Nursing intervention and treatment
• Adjust material to the nature and severity of the retraction
• Consider using a convex skin barrier, possibly supplemented by padding and not too tight fitting support belt(2, 7, 13)
• If there is no solution in terms of adequate stoma material, surgical revision should be considered (2, 3, 7, 27).

Stoma stenosis
Definition
Impairment of effluent drainage due to narrowing or contraction of the stomal tissue at the level of the skin or fascia (2, 8, 27)

Incidence
Immediately postoperative (0.25%) to 10% in the post-clinical phase (27, 30)
Characteristics
• Explosive or narrow stools and loud flatus, pain during stoma production (2, 3, 7)
• In urostomy, pain in the flank, decreased urine production or projectile emptying of urine from high residuals of urine in the bowel loop, dark and foul-smelling urine resulting in repeated urinary tract infections (2, 3, 7, 27)
Cause and Risk Factors
• Surgical operation technique (2, 7) inadequate positioning in the fascia layer or insufficient loosening of the skin layers (2)
• Prior radiation to the bowel segment (2)
• Urostomy (27)
• Excessive scar forming around the stoma (2, 3, 7)
• Recurring carcinoma (7)
Consequences
• Complaints of obstruction (2)
• Complete blockage of the stoma (3)
Nursing intervention and treatment
• Check by touching the dimension and the flexibility of the skin and fascial ring (7). If this is not possible, refer to surgeon.
• Try to keep the stool supple by increased fluid intake and use of medication (2, 3, 7)
• Dilating the stoma with a special dilator by nurse or patient. Although controversial since the stenosis may worsen by formation of scar tissue caused by dilation (2, 3, 7, 27).
• In severe stenosis surgical intervention may be required (7, 27).

Stoma trauma
Definition
Laceration of stomal mucosa often because of pressure or physical force (8)
Incidence
Unknown
Characteristics
• Yellow or white discoloration of the stomal mucosa (2)
• Defect, which easily bleeds (2)
• Often not painful, problem is noticed when stoma is managed (2)
Cause and Risk Factors
• Stoma rubs against stoma appliance because of a poor fit or use of a belt (2)
• Prolapsed stoma (2)
• Parastomal hernia (2)
• Trauma by accident (2)
Consequences
• Oedema
• Bleeding stoma
• Necrosis
Nursing intervention and treatment
• Eliminate the causative factor, adjust stoma care appliance to stoma shape and size (2)
• If necessary, stop the bleeding

Stoma fistula
Definition
An abnormal communication between the stoma and the surrounding tissue or in the stoma other than the lumen (8)
Incidence
Unknown

Characteristics
Stool is discharged from the body from unnatural places other than the stoma but in the immediate vicinity of the stoma
Cause and Risk Factors
• Too deep suturing (through the different tissue layers) in stoma construction
• Crohn's disease
Consequences
• Leakage
• Erosion of the peristomal skin
Nursing intervention and treatment
Customize stoma appliances

PERISTOMAL PROBLEMS

Contact Dermatitis
Definition
Skin damage through contact with faeces, urine or chemical preparations (8)
Incidence
• from 10% to 43% (39)
• Redness of the skin or rash around the stoma 26% (36)
• More prevalent in ileostomy or colostomy at 30-40% (43)
• More prevalent in ileostomy and urostomy especially in strong acidic or alkaline urine (3)
Characteristics
• Red skin and moist, erosion, painful, localized to the region of contact (38)
• Skin irritation (3, 22)
Cause and Risk Factors
• Leakage (3, 22, 26)
• Not properly fitted stoma appliance (38)
• Removing stoma appliances incorrectly (3)
Consequences
• Insufficient adhesion of stoma appliance
• leakage
Nursing intervention and treatment
• Identify the cause and adjust stoma appliance (3, 43)
• Make use of stoma accessories
• Referral to dermatologist for treatment with topical corticosteroid (emulsion or lotion)

Granuloma
Definition
Excessive tissue occurring at the skin/stoma base in areas of retained or reactive suture material (8)
Incidence
2% of stomal problems (18)
Characteristics
• Raspberry like growth (8)
• Pain
• Fast bleeding, haemorrhages (3, 27)
Causes and Risk Factors
• Repeated trauma (by stoma appliance) or chronic contact with faeces (3, 25)
• Reaction to suture material (8)
Consequences
Insufficient adhesion of stoma appliance causing leakage

Nursing intervention and treatment
• Dab with silver nitrate (3, 27) or apply pressure (convex skin barrier) (19)
• Ask physician in a consultation to exclude malignancy/viral infection (3)
• Refer to dermatologist for cryotherapy

Candidiasis
Definition
An overgrowth of fungal organisms (Candida) sufficient to cause infection of the skin around the stoma (25)
Incidence
unknown
Characteristics
•Red rash, white flaking, sometimes small papules and itching, clear marking (38)
Causes and Risk Factors
• Warm, dark and damp places (e.g. underneath the skin barrier) (33)
• Repeated use of antibiotics (25)
• Diabetes Mellitus
• Lowered resistance
Consequences
Difficult stoma management and leakage
Nursing intervention and treatment
• medication, local application (on physician's orders), preferably spray or powder (25)
• Adjust stoma appliance if necessary
• Ask dermatologist in consultation to consider oral therapy or culture

Folliculitis
Definition
Inflammation of hair follicle of the peristomal skin (8)
Incidence
Unknown
Characteristics
•Erythema with pustules around the hair follicle and papillae
Causes and Risk Factors (22, 25)
• Staphylococcus aureus, Streptococci, or a combination of the two (8, 25)
• Careless shaving the peristomal skin
• Removing stoma appliance harshly
• Prolonged use of topical corticosteroids
Result
Pain and itching
Nursing intervention and treatment
Adjusting stoma care

Pseudo verrucous lesions
Definition
Wart-like lesions in the peristomal area caused by chronic exposure to moisture and irritation (8)
Incidence
Unknown
Characteristics
• Skin around stoma looks softened (maceration) and is thickened
• can occur with or without crystal forming
Causes and Risk Factors
• Chronic effects of moisture
• Unsuitable stoma material (38)
• In flushing and stoma retraction (38)

Result

Local pain, leakage

Nursing intervention and treatment

• Dab the lesion with a silver nitrate pen

• Adjust stoma care appliance so that skin lesions are covered.

• More frequent exchange of appliance, possibly convex collecting material.

• Apply compress with acetic acid aqueous solution of 5% on the skin for several minutes.

Pyoderma gangrenosum

Definition

An ulcerative skin condition of unknown etiology occurring around the stoma (8)

Incidence

Rare. 1-5% in patients with IBD (32)

Characteristics

•Very painful, heaved red skin around skin ulceration with skin lesions, jagged subverted wound edges, bluish discolouring.

Causes and Risk Factors

Unknown (3, 38), sometimes associated with IBD and rheumatism

Result

Ulcerative skin lesions and leakage (3)

Nursing intervention and treatment

• Given the extreme course, early diagnosis and multidisciplinary treatment is essential (15)

• Medication, oral and local (15) ordered by physician

• Appropriate stoma appliance (3)

• Adequate wound management to absorb the moisture(38)

Stoma varices (Caput medusae)

Definition

Large portosystemic venous collateral blood vessels that are visible next to the stoma(8)

Incidence

Unknown

Characteristics

• Purple discoloration by dilated, meandering veins around the stoma (38)

• Bleeding of the mucocutaneous edge of stoma (41)

Cause and Risk Factors

Portal hypertension due to liver cirrhosis

Result

Insufficient adhesion of stoma appliance due to bleeding or changed skin texture

Nursing intervention and treatment

• Refer to a physician on short term in connection with diagnosis and underlying suffering (38)

• Stop bleeding (local pressure with icy wet gauze)

• Appropriate stoma appliance, careful pressure

• Remove stoma appliance carefully without tension on the skin

OTHER PROBLEMS at the stoma

Leakage

Definition

Stool or urine that penetrates between the skin barrier and the skin, as a result of a complication or other problem.

Incidence

0-62% (17, 24, 35, 36)

Cause and Risk Factors
• Urostomy or ileostomy (21)
• Poorly constructed stoma (38)
• Poor stoma siting (2, 35)
• Unevenness around stoma caused by skin fold, indentation or scars
• Improper stoma care (9, 17, 34, 35, 38)
• Skin disorders (18)
• Increasing or decreasing of waist circumference, (17, 38)
• Stoma complications
• Receiving chemotherapy and radiotherapy (21)
Result
• psychosocial problems (17, 18, 24, 28, 36, 35, 42,)
• Peristomal skin disorders (18)
• Problematic stoma care
• More appliances usage
Nursing intervention
Identify and eliminate the cause of leakage or eliminate the effect thereof.

Pancaking
Definition
Pancaking occurs when the faeces does not move down into the stoma bag, but remains around the stoma (3)
Incidence
Unknown
Cause and Risk Factors
• The consistency of the stool can be too thick or sticky.
• The stoma bag draws a vacuum.
• Usually in colostomies (3)
Result
• Stool pushes the skin barrier away from the skin.
• Leakage
Nursing intervention and treatment
• Advice regarding fluid intake and nutrition
• Prevent vacuuming
• Lubricant in the bag
• Adjust stoma appliance

Oedema
Definition
Accumulation of fluid in the stoma causing the stoma to enlarge
Incidence
Unknown
Cause and Risk Factors
• Postoperative (2, 14, 42)
• Appliance cut too tight/wrong material
• Stoma prolaps (2)
• Oedema elsewhere in the body
• Increased intra-abdominal pressure
• Stoma obstruction
• Irritation of mucosa
Result
• Can complicate stoma management
• Stoma necrosis (2)

Nursing intervention
• Adjust stoma appliance (38)
• Cold gauze (2)
• Powdered sugar (2)
• Use Xylometazoline spray after consultation with physician

COMPLICATIONS RELATED TO STOOL PATTERN

<u>**High output in bowel stoma**</u>
Definition
Stoma production from a bowel stoma of more than 1 litre per 24 hours (40)
Incidence
Unknown
Cause and Risk Factors
• Ileostomy or stoma situated on an even higher part of the intestine. Therefore functional length of small intestine (14, 40)
• Postoperative after bowel surgery (14, 40)
• Intestine illness e.g. Crohn's disease (40), bowel infections, bowel failure (40)
• Antibiotics
• Chemotherapy
Consequences
• Watery loose stools and difficulty to regulate production with intake of food and fluids (40)
• Dehydration
• Electrolyte imbalance
• Problems with collecting and leakage
• Unreliable oral contraceptives.
Nursing intervention
• Referral to specialist
• Fluid and dietary measures (4, 14, 40) See Appendix XII
• Refer to dietician
• Monitoring fluid balance
• Adjust stoma appliance (40) with ample capacity.

<u>**Obstruction (ileus)**</u>
Definition
Blockage of the stomal passage resulting in no stool and/or flatus
Incidence
Unknown
Cause and Risk factors
• Food plug (for risky foods, see Appendix XII)
• The passage of bowel part through fascia and muscle layer (12)
• The slimmer bowel lumen of an ileostomy. (12)
• Stomal complication such as parastomal hernia and/or stenosis
• Postoperative after bowel surgery
• Obstipation
• Carcinoma in bowel lumen
• Mechanical or paralytic ileus
• Bowel perforation
Consequences
• Reduced or absence of flatus
• Nausea and (faecal) vomiting
• Swollen or oedematous stoma, abdominal distension
• Restlessness

• Abdominal cramps with paradoxical diarrhoea or no stool at all
Nursing intervention
• Immediate referral to specialist
• Stop food intake, but if possible ample fluid intake (6)
• If ordered by a physician: flushing in ileostomy, clyster or irrigation in colostomy

Obstipation
Definition
Accumulation of faeces in the colon, resulting in a delayed excretion of hard, dry stools through the stoma (5)
Incidence
Unknown
Cause and Risk Factors
• Food with too little fibre and moisture
• Not properly chewed food
• Underlying disease with impaired peristalsis
• Incomplete (bowel) obstruction
• Medical treatment or diagnosis
• Medication: opiates, anti-depressants, iron supplements, laxatives etc.
• Inactivity
Consequences
• Change in frequency and consistency of stools (pattern)
• Dry/swollen mucosa
• Full feeling in the abdomen, abdominal distension
• Excessive gas forming
• Poor appetite, nausea
• Pain before defecation, abdominal cramps
• Obstruction and ileus
• More likely in obstipation: prolapse, parastomal hernia, retraction and stenosis (hard stools can cause tissue rupture and scarring, resulting in stenosis).
Nursing intervention
• Lifestyle, fluid and nutritional recommendations (see Appendix XII)
• Refer to dietician
• Medication prescribed by a physician
• Bowel irrigation after consulting physician (5)

Excessive gas forming
Definition
Gas forming to such an extent that the ostomate feels constrained.
Incidence
Unknown
Cause and Risk Factors
• Colostomy (5)
• Abnormalities of the bowel flora (5)
• Swallowing air by smoking, talking while eating, chewing gum (3)
• Certain foods (3) (see Appendix XII)
• Obstipation
• Stomal complications such as parastomal hernia and stenosis
Consequences
• Visibility of stoma appliance caused by ballooning
• Noise and odour

Nursing intervention
• Advice in regard with fluid intake and nutrition (3) (see Appendix XII)
• Modifications of appliance regarding odour and filters
• Teach bowel irrigation (3)

Article	Level	Nr in Appendix
Arumugam, P.J., Bevan, L., Macdonald, L., Watkins, A.J., Morgan, A.R., Beynon, J., Carr, ND (2003). A prospective audit of stoma analysis of riskfactors and complications. *Colorectal disease, 5,* 49-52.	C	1
Barr, J.E. (2004). Assessment and management of stomal complications: a framework for clinical decision making. Os*tomy wound manage, 50(9),* 50- 67.	D	2
Burch, J. (2005 a). Stoma complications encountered in the community, AZ. *British Journal of community nursing, 10(7),* 324-329.	D	3
Burch, J. (2006). Nutrition and the ostomate: input, output and absorption. *British journal of community nursing, 11(8),* 349-351.	D	4
Burch, J. (2007). Obstipation and flatulence management for stoma patients. *British journal of community nursing, 12(10),* 449-452.	D	5
Burch, J. (2008 a). Nutrition for people with stomas. 2: An overview of dietary advice. *Nursing times, 104(49),* 26-27. www.nursingtimes.net.	D	6
Butler, D.L. (2009). Early postoperative complications following ostomy surgery: a review. *Journal of wound ostomy continence nursing, 36(5),* 513-519.	C	7
Colwell, J.C. & Beitz, J., (2007 a). Survey of wound, ostomy and continence (WOC) nurse clinicians on stomal and peristomal complications: a content validation study. *Journal of wound ostomy continence nursing, 34(1),* 57-69.	C	8
Colwell, J.C. & Gray, M. (2007b). Does preoperative teaching and stoma site marking affect surgical outcomes in patients undergoing ostomy surgery? *Journal of wound ostomy continence nursing, 34(5),* 492-496.	C	9
Cottam, J., Richards, A., Hasted, A., Blackman, A. (2006). Results of a nationwide prospective audit of stoma complications within 3 weeks of surgery. *Colorectal disease, 9,* 834-838. doi: 10.1111/j.1463-1318.2007.01213. *x*	C	10
De Raet, J., Delvaux, G., Haentjens, P., Van Nieuwenhove, Y. (2008). Waist circumference is an independent risk factor for the development of parastomal hernia after permanent colstomy. *Diseases of the colon & rectum, 51,* 1806–1809. doi: 10.1007/s10350-008-9366-5	C	11
Doughty, D. (2005). Principles of ostomy management in oncology patients. *The journal of supportive oncology, 3(1),* 59-69.	D	12
Fulham, J. (2008 a). A guide to caring for patients with a newly formed stoma in the acute hospital setting. *Gastrointestinal nursing, 6(8),* 14-23.	D	13
Fulham, J. (2008 b).Providing dietary advice for the individual with a stoma. *British journal of nursing, 17(2),* 22-27.	D	14
Funayama, Y., Kumagai, E., Takahashi, K.I., Fukushima, K., Sasaki, I. (2009). Early diagnosis and early corticosteroid administration improves healing of peristomal pyoderma gangrenosum in inflammatory bowel disease. *Diseases of the colon & rectum, 52(2),* 311-314. doi:10.1007/DCR.0b013e31819accc6	B	15
Gray, M., Colwell, J.C., Goldberg, M.T. (2005). What treatments are effective for the management of peristomal hernia? *Journal of wound ostomy continence nursing, 32 (2) ,* 87-92.	B	16
Haugen, V., Bliss, DZ, Savik, K. (2006). Perioperative factors that affect long-term adjustment to an incontinent ostomy. *Journal of wound ostomy continence nursing, 33(5),* 525-535.	B	17

Herlufsen, P., Olsen, A.G., Carlsen, B., Nybaek, H., Karlsmark, T., Laursen, T.N., Jemec, G.B.E. (2006). OstomySkin study: a study of peristomal skin disorders in patients with permanent stomas. *British journal of nursing, 15(16)*, 854-862.	C	18
Johnson, S. (2007). Tape for the treatment of overgranulation tissue. *Wounds UK, product review, 3(3)*.	D	19
Kald, A., Juul, K.N., Hjortsvang, H., Sjödahl, R.I.(2008). Quality of life is impaired in patients with peristomal bulging of a sigmoid colostomy. *Scandinavian journal of gastroenterology, 43*, 627-633. doi:10.1080/00365520701858470	C	20
Nederlandse Stomavereniging (2009a). *Stomagerelateerde complicaties. Onderzoeksverslag in opdracht van de NSV* . Amsterdam: Newcom Research & Consultancy B.V. Kapteijns, A. & Buitinga, S.	C	21
Kouba, E., Sands, M., Lentz, A., Wallen, E., Pruthi, R.S. (2007). Incidence and Risk Factors of stomal complications in patients undergoing cystectomy with ileal conduit urinary diversion for bladder cancer. *The journal of urology, 178,*950-954. doi:10.1016/j.juro.2007.05.028	C	23
Lynch, B.M., Hawkes A.L., Steginga S.K., Leggett B., Aitken, J.F. (2008). Stoma surgery for colorectal cancer. A population-based study of patient concerns. *Journal of wound ostomy continence nursing, 35(4)*, 424-428.	C	24
Lyon, C.C. & Smith, A.J. (2001). Abdominal stomas and their skin disorders. An atlas of diagnosis and management. *Martin Dunitz, London*, ISBN 1-85317-896-9.	D	25
Lyon, C.C., Smith, A.J., Griffiths, C.E.M., Beck, M.H. (2000). The spectrum of skin disorders in abdominal stoma patients. *British journal of dermatology, 143*, 1248-1260.	C	26
Nazarko, L. (2008). Caring for a patient with a urostomy in a community setting. *British journal of community nursing, 13(8)*, 354-361.	D	27
Nordström, G.M. & Nyman, C.R. (1991). Living with a urostomy. A follow up with special regard to the peristomal-skin complications, psychosocial and sexual life. *Scandinavian journal of Urol. Nephrol. Suppl., 138*, 247-251.	C	28
Nybaek, H., Bang Knudsen, D., Norgaard Laursen, T., Karlsmark, T.J., Jemec, G.B.E. (2 009).Skin problems in ostomy patients: a case-control study of risk factors. *Acta derm venereol, 89*, 64-67. doi:10.2340/00015555-0536	C	29
Park, J.J., Del Pino, A., Orsay, C.P., Nelson, RL, Pearl, L.K., Cintron, J.R., Abcarian, H. (1999). Stoma complications: the Cook County Hospital experience. *Diseases of the colon & rectum, 42(12)*, 1575-1580.	C	30
Pilgrim, C.H.C., McIntyre, R., Bailey, M. (2010). Prospective audit of parastomal hernia: prevalence and associated comorbidities. *Diseases of the colon & rectum, 53(1)*, 71–76. doi: 10.1007/DCR.0b013e3181bdee8c	B	31
Poritz, L.S., Lebo, MA, Bobb, A.D., Ardell, C.M., Koltun, W.A. (2008). Management of peristomal pyoderma gangrenosum. *Journal of the American college of surgeons, 206*, 311–315. doi:10.1016/j.jamcollsurg.2007.07.023	C	32
Ratliff, C.R. & Donovan, A.M. (2001). Frequency of peristomal complications. O*stomy wound management, 47(8)*, 26-29.	C	33
Readding, L.A. (2005). Hospital to home, smoothing the journey for the new ostomist. *British journal of nursing, 14(16)*, 16-20.	D	34
Redmond, C., Cowin, C., Parker, T. (2009).The experience of faecal leakage among ileostomists. *British journal of nursing, 18(17)*, 12-17.	C	35
Richbourg, L., Thorpe, J.M., Rapp, C.G. (2007). Difficulties experienced by the ostomate after hospital discharge. *Journal of wound ostomy continence nursing, 34 (1)*, 70-79.	C	36
PON (2006). *Parastomale hernia en hulpmiddelengebruik* . Tilburg: PON	D	37

Rietveld, T. & Erp, S. van		
Rolstad, B.S. & Erwin-Toth, P.L. (2010). Peristomal skin complications: prevention and management. *American journal of nursing, 110 (2),* 43-48.	D	38
Salvadalena, G. (2008). Incidence of complications of the stoma and peristomal skin among individuals with colostomy, ilestomy, and urstomy: a systematic review. *Journal of wound ostomy continence nursing, 3 5(6),* 596-607.	C	39
Sica, J. & Burch, J. (2007). Management of bowel failure and high-output stomas. *British journal of nursing, 16(13),* 772- 777.	D	40
Spier, B.J., Fayyad, A.A., Lucey, M.R., Johnson, E.A., Wojtowycz, M., Rikkers, H., Harms, B.A., Reichelderfer, M. (2008). Bleeding stomal varices: case series and systematic review of the literature. *Clinical gastroenterology and hepatology, 6,* 346-352. doi: 10.1016/j.cgh.2007.12.047	C	41
Vujnovich, A. (2008) Pre and post- operative assessment of patients with a stoma. *Nursing standard, 22(19),* 50-56.	D	42
Woo, K.Y., Sibbald, R.G., Ayello, E.A., Coutts, P.M., Garde, D.E. (2009). Peristomal Skin Complications and Management. Advanced in skin & wound care, 22(11), 522-532.	D	22
Yeo,H., Abir, F., Longo, WE (2006). Management of parastomal ulcers. *World Journal of Gastroenterology, 12(20),* 3133-3137.	D	43

Appendix XIV Transfer of the stoma care

General:
• Admission date and length of stay
• Diagnosis
• Treatment and/or type of operation
• Responsible physician/medical specialist

Stoma
• Date of stoma construction
• Type of stoma
• End/Loop/Temporary/Permanent

Progress/recovery treatment
• Physical/mental
• Social
• Expected after care

Description of the request for help to the community nurse or care institution
• Full help
• Support in learning stoma self-care
• Counselling

Stoma Care
• Did the ostomate have an informative consultation
• Description of details of the stoma
• Consistency and quantity of stoma production
• Details about sutures (soluble yes/no)/bridge/splints
• Diameter of the stoma, measurements of the opening of the skin barrier, offer a template
• Description of the peristomal skin
• Important aspects regarding stoma care
  o Date of previous stomal care:
  o Date of next stomal care:
• Extent of stomal selfcare
  o Independent
  o Need help with ......
  o Independent emptying
  o Stoma Care by spouse/community care/.......
reason:
• Specific points of attention .....

Choice of appliances and supplier:
• Item numbers of ordered stoma appliances and aids
• Phone numbers
• Delivery appointment

Outpatient check-up:
• Accessibility of the stoma care nurse
• Follow-up appointment with the stoma care nurse

Appendix XV
Information for the ostomate in the discharge phase and aftercare phase

The information in this Appendix has to be shared with the ostomate so that he will be aware of what is considered to be normal with regard to the stoma. In addition, practical issues for daily life are mentioned. This list might probably not be complete, but may be used in addition to the text in the guideline.

General observations of the stoma
• colour of the stomal mucosa: pink to bright red (similar to oral mucosa)
• shape: round/oval, height: between 5 mm and 20 mm above skin level (ideal situation)
• skin around the stoma same colour as the rest of the abdomen
• postoperative stoma is oedematous and shrinks in the first 8 weeks
• the mucous membrane of the stoma may easily bleed when touched (for cleaning), and if anti-coagulant medication is used

Description of the output
• **Colostomy and ileostomy:**
Depending on the location of the stoma, and when the patient has resumed normal eating and drinking, the stool pattern will be as follows:
  o stoma on the ileum: (watery)thin to gruel-like stool, several times per day
  o stoma on the ascending colon, thin to gruel-like stools several times a day
  o stoma on the transverse section, gruel-like stool, two to three times per day
  o stoma on the descending colon, firm stools, once or twice a day, sometimes
  skipping a day
• Urostomy:
The urine should have a clear colour, mixed with some mucus (from the ileum loop). 1200ml to 1500 ml of urine will be produced by the urostomy per 24 hours.
With high fever and back pain, the urostomate is advised to contact the doctor/medical specialist the same day because of increased risk of urinary tract infections or kidney infections. When a urine culture is required in a urostomy, the urine should be taken directly from the stoma. The urine in the urostomy bag contains microorganisms and does not provide correct results.

Excessive hair growth around the stoma
In case of excessive hair growth on the abdomen, the skin around the stoma can be shaved with a disposable blade. It is advisable to shave away from the stoma. Hygiene is important to prevent small wounds. After shaving, barrier cream may be applied to the skin. In extreme hair growth, the ostomate can be referred to a dermatologist to discuss the possibility of laser treatment. Be cautious with using substances such as hair removers because of a possible reaction to the parastomal skin.

Physical labour

Lifting

Ostomates are advised against lifting objects the first six to eight weeks after surgery and then to gradually build up labour and activities. Ensure that lifting is done in a proper way, with minimal stress on the abdomen and especially the abdominal muscles. Heavy objects (more than ten to fifteen kilograms) should not be lifted at all because this causes too much pressure on the abdominal muscles.

Sports

Ostomates can participate in many sports but during the first eight to twelve weeks intensive sports are advised against. In those weeks the stoma has still to form its permanent size and shape. After that period, if necessary, protective belts and caps can be used.

Endurance sports or heavy physical exertion require some adjustment with an ileostomy and urostomy. Ileostomates must ensure adequate fluid intake. Often extra salt intake is also necessary. In endurance sports the urostomy and ileostomy often produce less. Sports that should rather not be exercised with a stoma are: weightlifting, power-intensive contact sports such as rugby, judo, karate and wrestling.

Leaflets describing abdominal exercises suitable for ostomates are available.

Swimming and sauna

It is possible to swim with a stoma. The stoma appliance should not be placed shortly before swimming, since the adhesive strength is not yet optimal. The filter can be covered with a patch to protect it against water. There are also filter membranes to prevent water from getting into the carbon filter of the bag without preventing gas emission. Smaller bags may be used when swimming. Special swimwear is available and there are companies who custom-make swimsuits.

It is possible to visit the sauna with a stoma. Stoma patches are available to cover the stoma.

Work

Having a stoma is not a reason in itself to be unable to work.

Travelling and Holiday

When on holiday or travelling, it is important to take along sufficient supplies of stoma material (Advice: one and a half to twice the normal amount) Due to temperature differences and change of diet, the consumption of appliances may be higher. Pack the stoma appliances in various bags and hand baggage in case the luggage gets lost.

Stoma Passport

Stoma passports are available from the stoma care nurse, the Dutch Ostomy Association or medical specialist shops. This can be very useful for travelling abroad. All the information that customs officers or security might need, is presented in several languages in the stoma passport.

Warm weather

When it is hot, extra fluid intake is important to avoid dehydration (minimum 1, 5 litres of water per day). Ileostomates should increase both fluid and salt intake.

Water

If the water is not fit to drink, it is better to buy bottled water. Take note that the bottles are sealed. Bottled water should even be used for stoma irrigation because the bowel also absorbs water.

Stoma word list

There are brochures available which contain the most important questions and answers related to ostomy in all European languages.

Thickening agents

Situations can occur where the use of thickening agents might prove more comfortable to the ostomate. These agents are placed in the bag to thicken the output.

Appendix XVI   Description of stoma appliances and accessories

	Generic categories	Description	Indications	Contra-indications/ warnings
1	Stoma system	**One-piece:** Skin barrier and bag form a unit. With each change the bag with adhesive layer is removed from the skin	Ostomate's preference Construction and shape of the stoma Dexterity and vision Physical activities	
		Two-piece: Combination of skin barrier and changeable stoma bags	Ostomate's preference Skin condition Pain Exchange various stoma bags	
2	Skin barrier	**Composition:** Natural materials Synthetic polymers **Shape:** Plane Spherical	Protecting peristomal skin

Stomal retraction | Postoperative Parastomal hernia |
| | | **Contours:** Round Square Oval Flower shaped **Opening:** Fit to cut Pliable Mouldable Pre-formed | Ostomate's preference and Build

Dexterity and ostomate's preference Stoma shape | Oval stoma |
| | | **Connection:** Click Adhesive **Flange:** Stationary Floating **Fixing:** Without patch edge With patch edge | Ostomate's dexterity and vision Ostomate's preference Ostomate's preference and dexterity

Skin conditions Fixing of skin barrier | Skin conditions |
| 3 | Stoma bag/cap | **Closed** **Open:** Integrated fastening Tap Fastening clip **Collecting capacity:** | Stool consistency Ileo-/urostomy Ostomate's preference and dexterity

Production/ostomate's preference/build | |

		Appearance:		
		Transparent	Observing stoma/output	
		View port	Ostomate's preference	
		Opaque		
		Anatomic/symmetrical	Build/ostomate's preference	
		Partitioned	Urostomy	
		Filter	Odourless emission of bowel gases	Leakage through filter
		Flushable	Ostomate's preference	
4	Fillers	**Paste disks:**	Filling up folds and pits	
		Round/oval	Prevent leakage	
		Mouldable/pre-formed		
		Convex		
		Pastes:		
		With alcohol		
		Without alcohol		Peristomal dermatitis
		Strips		
		Wedge		
		Hydrocolloid mouldable ring		
5	Powder	Absorption of moisture	Peristomal skin damage	Adhesion of skin barrier
		Protection		
6	Skin protection	Cream	Care/protection	
		Film	Protection against aggressive output	
7	Fixatives	Adhesive strips of various materials and shapes	Increasing the adhesive surface of skin barrier	
		Adhesive spray	Extra adhesion	
8	Belt	Belt for extra support for appliance	Extra support	
9	Supportive binder	Various models and sizes	Parastomal hernia and prolapse	Careful in convexity
10	Lubricant	Lubricant in bag	Pancaking	
11	Binding agent	Capsules	Thickening of stool	
		Tablets		
		Sachets		
		Strips		
12	Odour neutralizers	Sachets	Reduces odour	
		Drops		
13	Stoma dilator	Conical or tapered rod	Treatment of stenosis on skin or fascia level of stoma	
14	Adhesive removers	Tissue	Remove adhesive layer	Reduce adhesion
		Spray		
15	Stoma irrigation accessories	Flush bags, flush pump, cone, sleeves	Irrigation	Colostomy only
16	Stoma patch	Provides protection and isolation	After irrigation and in continent stoma	
17	Stoma sealing system	Various types	Continence	Colostomy only
18	Night drainage/leg bag	Extra collecting capacity	Urostomy/high output ileostomy	

Appendix XVII   Specific stoma care tasks with associated skills levels

Treating complications, establishing policy	Stoma care nurse
Removing bridge	Stoma care nurse
Removing necrotic tissue from the stoma	Stoma care nurse
Teach irrigation	Stoma care nurse
Locating stoma site	level 4 and 5 skilled nurse or stoma care nurse
Flushing and irrigating the stoma	Level 4 and 5 nurses
Administering medication via the stoma	Level 4 and 5 nurses
Dilating the stoma	Level 4 and 5 nurses
Internal examination of the stoma	Level 4 and 5 nurses
Remove sutures	Level 4 and 5 nurses
Applying silver nitrate	Level 4 and 5 nurses
Treating complications, executing established policy	Level 4 and 5 nurses
Teaching self-care	Level 4 and 5
Changing one-piece and two-piece stoma appliance in uncomplicated stoma care	From level 3
Identifying complications	From level 3

The general rule of competence and jurisdiction applies to all these tasks.

Appendix XVIII Patient Information

Nederlandse Stomavereniging; The Dutch Ostomy Association
The Dutch Ostomy Association aims to promote the best possible physical, mental and social condition of people with a stoma or pouch and people who had a stoma.
Address: Bison Staete 1230 Bisonspoor 3605 KZ Maarssen
Phone: (0346) 26 22 86
Website: www.stomavereniging.nl

SPKS
Foundation for Patients with Cancer of the Digestive Tract is a patient organization for cancer patients, their spouses and their immediate environment. SPKS facilitates contact between these parties and represents their interests.
Address: Secretariat SPKS
c/o Dutch Federation of Cancer Organizations (NFK)
PO Box 8152 3503 RD Utrecht
Phone: 0800 022 66 22
Website: http://www.spks.nfk.nl

Crohn's and Colitis Ulcerosa Association (CCUVN)
The Crohn's and Colitis Association of the Netherlands (CCUVN) is committed to people with Crohn's disease and colitis ulcerosa and related disorders. The CCUVN provides information, facilitates support groups and represents the interests of patients.
Address: 4 Houttuinlaan 3447 GM Woerden
Phone: (0348) 420780
Website: www.crohn-colitis.nl and www.ccjongeren.nl

The Dutch Digestive Foundation (Mdl)
The Dutch Digestive Foundation is committed on several fronts for stomach, liver and intestine patients. They fund important research into diseases of the digestive system.
Address: 95 Stationsplein 3818 LE Amersfoort
Phone: 0900-2025625
Website: www.mlds.nl

Interstitial Cystitis Patient Association (ICP)
The Interstitial Cystitis Patient Association represents the interests of people with IC and the bladder pain syndrome. It does so by providing information to patients, promote scientific research and provide contact with a support group. The ICP has a medical advisory board of experts in the field of interstitial cystitis.
Address: PO Box 4 3980 CA Bunnik
Phone: (030) 296 29 6
Website: www.icpatienten.nl

The Foundation for Pelvic floor Patients (SBP)
(De Stichting Bekkenbodem Patiënten (SBP))

The Foundation for Pelvic floor Patients (SBP) is an association dedicated to people with pelvic floor complaints. SBP does this by providing information on complaints as a result of decreased function of the pelvic floor.

Address: PO Box 183 2950 AD Alblasserdam

Phone: (020) 6586520

Website: www.bekkenbodem.net

Dutch Association of Hirschsprung Disease

The Association of Hirschsprung Disease is a patient association, where patients, parents/guardians or other interested parties can meet with peers.

Address: c/o 34 Mezenstraat 1223 PH Hilversum

Phone: (035) 685 60 15/ (078) 6918687

Website: www.hirschsprung.nl

Irritable Bowel Syndrome (IBS) Interest Group

The purpose of the Irritable Bowel Syndrome Interest Group (PDSB) is to support people with IBS in living with the disease, by facilitating contact with support groups, providing patients, doctors and others with information, promoting research on the causes and treatment of IBS, improving treatment and care and represent the interests of patients.

Address: PO Box 2597 8901 AB Leeuwarden

Phone: PDS info line: (088) 737 4636

Website: www.pdsb.nl

Polyposis Contact Group (PPC)

PPC is an association committed to people with Polyposis Coli, a hereditary syndrome that causes polyp formation in the bowel, and in many cases causes bowel cancer. The syndrome is also known under the name of Familial Adomateuze Polyposis, abbreviated FAP

Address: 5 Muntslagererf 6043 SM Roermond

Phone: (0475) 328720

Website: www.polyposis.nl

Patient organization for Anal-rectal Malformation

This is a national patient organization that aims to represent the interests of people who are born with anus atresia and their parents.

Address: PO Box 78 1270 AB Huizen

Phone: (035) 5233782

Website: www.anusatresie.nl

HNPCC Association (Hereditary non-polyposis colorectal cancer)
The purpose of the association is to bring patients with HNPCC-Lynch syndrome and others who are involved, in contact with each other. The association aims to optimally represent patients' interests and to support the patients with dealing with the effects of the disease.
Address: c/o NFK PO Box 8152 3503 RD Utrecht
Phone: (0800) 022 66 22
Website: www.kankerpatient.nl/hnpcc

Waterloop Association
Patients have questions before, during and after treatment. Not everyone has someone close to share their feelings with. For this reason the Association Waterloop was established.
Address: c/o NFK PO Box 8152 3503 RD Utrecht
Phone: (030)-2916090
Website: www.kankerpatient.nl/waterloop

KWF Dutch Cancer Society
Mission: Reducing cancer and getting it under control. We are there for people living with cancer and the people who live with them.
Address: 17 Delflandavenue 1062 EA Amsterdam
Phone: (020) 5700500
Website: http://www.kwfkankerbestrijding.nl

Stomaatje.nl
Website with all the ins & outs of stoma
Website: http://www.stomaatje.nl

REFERENCE LIST

	Level
Aiken, L.H., Clarke, S.P., Cheung, R.B., Sloane D.M. & Silber, J.H. (2003). Educational levels of hospital nurses and surgical patient mortality. *JAMA. 290(12),* 1617- 23.	B
Arumugam, P.J., Bevan, L., Macdonald, L., Watkins, A.J., Morgan, A.R., Beynon, J. & Carr, N.D. (2003). A prospective audit of stoma analysis of riskfactors and complications. *Colorectal Disease, 5(1),* 49-52.	C
ASCRS and WOCN Society (2007). Joint position statement on the value of preoperative stoma. Marking for patients undergoing fecal ostomy surgery. *Journal of Wound, Ostomy and Continence Nursing, 34(6),* 627-8.	D
Aukamp, V. & Sredl, D. (2004) Collaborative care management for a pregnant woman with an ostomy. *Complementary Therapy in Nursing & Midwifery, 10(1),* 5-12. doi:10.1016/S1353-6117(03)00077-5.	D
Barr, J.E. (2004). Assessment and management of stomal complications: a framework for clinical decision making. *Ostomy Wound Manage, 50(9),* 50- 67.	D
Bass, E.M., Del Pino, A., Tan, A., Pearl, R.K., Orsay, C.P. & Abcarian, H. (1997). Does preoperative stoma marking and education by the enterostomal therapist affect outcome? *Diseases of the Colon & Rectum, 40(4),* 440-442.	B
Black, P.K. (2004). Psychological, sexual and cultural issues for patients with a stoma. *British Journal of Nursing, 13(12),* 692-697.	D
Blegen, M.A., Vaughn, T.E. & Goode, C.J. (2001). Nurse Experience and Education: Effect on Quality of Care. *The Journal of Nursing Administration, 31(1),* 33-39.	B
Bosio, G. (2007). A proposal for classifying peristomale skin disorders: results of a multicenter observational study. *Ostomy Wound Manage. 53(9), 38-43.*	C
Brand, M.I. & Dujovny, N. (2008). Preoperative considerations and creation of normal ostomies. *Clinics in Colon and Rectal Surgery, 21(1),* 5-16.	D
Brown, H. & Randle, J. (2005). Living with a stoma: a review of the literature. *Journal of Clinical Nursing, 14(1),* 74-81.	B
Burch, J. (2005a). Stoma complications encountered in the community, A-Z. *British Journal of Community Nursing, 10(7),* 324-329.	D
Burch, J. (2005b). The pre- and postoperative nursing care for patients with a stoma. *British Journal of Nursing, 14(6),* 310-318.	D
Burch, J. (2006). Nutrition and the ostomate: input, output and absorption. *British Journal of Community Nursing, 11(8),* 349-351.	D
Burch, J. (2007). Obstipation and flatulence management for stoma patients. *British Journal of Community Nursing, 12(10),* 449-452.	D
Burch, J. (2008a). Nutrition for people with stomas. 2: An overview of dietary advice. *Nursing Times, 104(49),* 26-27.	D
Burch, J. (2008b). *Stomacare.* Chichester: John Wiley & Sons.	D
Butler, D.L. (2009). Early postoperative complications following ostomy surgery: a review. *Journal of Wound Ostomy Continence Nursing, 36(5),* 513-519.	C
Cataldo, P.A. (2008). Technical tips for stoma creation in the challenging patient. *Clinics in Colon and Rectal Surgery, 21(1),* 17-22.	D

Chaudhri, S., Brown, L., Hassan, H. & Horgan, A.F. (2005). Preoperative intensive, community-based vs. traditional stoma education: a randomized, controlled trial. *Diseases of the Colon & Rectum, 48(3),* 504-509.	B
Claessens- Spee, C.J., Geurts, E., Kessel v, I., Vink, M., Vliert v/d,N., (2001). Onderzoek naar de aard en incidentie van huidproblemen bij conventionele colo, ileo en/of urinestoma. *Rondom Stomazorg, 31,* 52-57.	C
Colwell, J.C. & Beitz, J., (2007). Survey of wound, ostomy and continence (WOC) nurse clinicians on stomal and peristomal complications: a content validation study. *Journal of Wound Ostomy Continence Nursing, 34(1),* 57-69.	C
Colwell, J.C. & Fichera, A. (2005). Care of the obese patient with an ostomy. *Journal of Wound Ostomy Continence Nursing, 32(6),* 378-383.	D
Colwell, J.C.& Gray, M. (2007). Does preoperative teaching and stoma site marking affect surgical outcomes in patients undergoing ostomy surgery? *Journal of Wound Ostomy Continence Nursing, 34(5),*492-496.	C
Cotrim, H. & Pereira, G. (2008). Impact of colorectal cancer on patient and family: implications for care. *European Journal of Oncology Nursing, 12(3),* 217- 226. doi: 10.1016/j.ejan.2007.11.005.	B
Cottam, J., Richards, A., Hasted, A. & Blackman, A. (2006). Results of a nationwide prospective audit of stoma complications within 3 weeks of surgery. *Colorectal Disease, 9(9),* 834-838. doi: 10.1111/j.1463-1318.2007.01213.x	C
De Gouveia Santos, V. L. C., Chaves, E.C. & Kimura, M. (2006). Quality of life and coping of persons with temporary and permanent stomas. *Journal of Wound Ostomy Continence Nursing, 33(5),* 503-509.	++
De Raet, J., Delvaux, G., Haentjens, P. & Van Nieuwenhove, Y. (2008). Waist circumference is an independent risk factor for the development of parastomal hernia after permanent colostomy. *Diseases of the Colon & Rectum, 51(12),* 1806–09. doi: 10.1007/s10350-008-9366-5	C
Doughty, D. (2005). Principles of ostomy management in oncology patients. *The Journal of Supportive Oncology, 3(1),* 59-69.	D
Duchesne, J.C., Wang, Y.Z., Weintraub, S.L., Boyle, M. & Hunt, J.P. (2002). Stoma complications: a multivariate analysis. *The American Surgeon, 68(11),* 961-968.	B
Erwin-Toth, P. (2006). Ostomy care and rehabilitation in colorectal cancer. *Seminars in Oncology Nursing, 22(3),* 174-177.	D
European Association of Urology Nurses (2009). *Good practice in health care: incontinent urostomy.* European Association of Urology Nurses Geng, V., Cobussen, H., Fillingham, S., Holroyd, S., Kiesbye, B. & Vahr, S.	AGREE
Fioravanti, M., Di Cesare, F., Ramelli, L., La Torre, F., Nicastro, A., Messinetti, S. & Lazzari, R. (1988). Pre-surgery information and psychological adjustment to enterostomy. *The Italian Journal of Surgical Science, 18(1),* 55-61.	C
Fleuren, M., Wieferink, K., & Paulussen, T. (2004). Determinants of innovation within healthcare organizations. Literature review and Delphi study. *International Journal for Quality in Health care, (16(2),* 107-123.	A
Fulham, J. (2008a). A guide to caring for patients with a newly formed stoma in the acute hospital setting. *Gastrointestinal Nursing, 6(8),* 14-23.	D
Fulham, J. (2008b).Providing dietary advice for the individual with a stoma. *British Journal of Nursing, 17(2),* 22-27.	D

Funayama, Y., Kumagai, E., Takahashi, K.I., Fukushima, K. & Sasaki, I. (2009). Early diagnosis and early corticosteroid administration improves healing of peristomal pyoderma gangrenosum in inflammatory bowel disease. *Diseases of the Colon & Rectum, 52(2),* 311-314. doi:10.1007/DCR.0b013e31819accc6.	B
Gallagher, S. & Gates, J. (2004). Challenges of ostomy care and obesity. *Ostomy Wound Management, 50(9),* 38-46.	D
Gray, M., Colwell, J.C. & Goldberg, M.T. (2005). What treatments are effective for the management of peristomal hernia? *Journal of Wound Ostomy Continence Nursing, 32(2),* 87-92.	B
Grol, R. & Wensing, M. (2006). *Implementatie. Effectieve verbetering van de patiëntenzorg.* Derde druk. Maarssen: Elsevier gezondheidszorg.	D
Haugen, V., Bliss, D.Z. & Savik, K. (2006). Perioperative factors that affect long-term adjustment to an incontinent ostomy. *Journal of Wound Ostomy Continence Nursing, 33(5),* 525-535.	B
Herlufsen, P., Olsen, A.G., Carlsen, B., Nybaek, H., Karlsmark, T., Laursen, T.N. & Jemec, G.B.E. (2006). OstomySkin study: a study of peristomal skin disorders in patients with permanent stomas. *British Journal of Nursing, 15(16),* 854-862.	C
Hunink, G. (1996). Onderzoeksverslagen lezen. *Tijdschrift voor Verpleegkundigen. 10,* 309-312.	D
Johnson, S. (2007). Tape for the treatment of overgranulation tissue. *Wounds UK, Product Review, 3(3).*	D
Junkin, J. & Beitz, J. (2005). Sexuality and the person with a stoma: Impliciations for comprehensive WOC nursing practice. *Journal of Wound Ostomy Continence Nursing, 32(2),* 121-128.	D
Kald, A., Juul, K.N., Hjortsvang, H.& Sjödahl, R.I. (2008). Quality of life is impaired in patients with peristomal bulging of a sigmoid colostomy. *Scandinavian Journal of Gastroenterology, 43(5),* 627-633. doi:10.1080/00365520701858470.	C
Karadaĝ, A., Menteş, B.B., & Ayaz S. (2004). Colostomy Irrigation: results of 25 cases with particular reference to quality of life. *Journal of Clinical Nursing, 14(4),* 479-485.	B
Karadaĝ, A., Menteş, B.B., Üner, A., İrKörücü, O., Ayaz, S. & Özkan, S. (2003). Impact of stomatherapy in quality of life in patients with permanent colostomies or ileostomies. *International Journal of Colorectal Disease, 18(3),* 234-238.	C
Kendall- Gallagher, D., Aiken, L.H., Sloane, D.M. & Cimiotti J.P. (2011). Nurse specialty certification, inpatient mortality, and failure to rescue. *Journal of Nursing scholarship, 43(2), 188-194.*	B
Kilic, E., Taycan, O., Belli, A.K. & Özmen, M. (2007). The effect of permanent ostomy on body image, self-esteem, marital adjustment, and sexual functioning. *Turkish Journal of Psychiatry, 18(4),* 1-8.	B
Klok, S.I. (2006). Uitwerking enquête raamwerk functie stomaverpleegkundige. *Rondom Stomazorg, 19(40),* 16-17.	D
Kouba, E., Sands, M., Lentz, A., Wallen, E. & Pruthi, R.S. (2007). Incidence and risk factors of stomal complications in patients undergoing cystectomy with ileal conduit urinary diversion for bladder cancer. *The Journal of Urology, 178(3),* 950-954. doi:10.1016/j.juro.2007.05.028.	C
Kuijpers, J.H.C. (2001). Gastro-intestinale chirurgie en gastro-enterologie. XI.	D

Stomata en stomachirurgie. *Nederlands Tijdschrift voor Geneeskunde, 145(24)*, 1144-48.	
Lo, SF., Wang, Y.T., Hsu, MY., Chang SC. & Hayter, M. (2009). A cost-effectiveness analysis of a multimedia learning education program for stoma patients. *Journal of Clinical Nursing, Epup: 4*,1-11. doi:10.1111/j.1365-2702.2009.02931.x.	B
Lynch, B.M., Hawkes A.L., Steginga S.K., Leggett B. & Aitken, J.F. (2008). Stoma surgery for colorectal cancer. A population-based study of patient concerns. *Journal of Wound Ostomy Continence Nursing, 35(4)*, 424-428.	C
Lyon, C.C. & Smith, A.J. (2001). *Abdominal stomas and their skin disorders. An atlas of diagnosis and management.* London: Martin Dunitz.	D
Lyon, C.C., Smith, A.J., Griffiths, C.E.M. & Beck, M.H. (2000). The spectrum of skin disorders in abdominal stoma patients. *British Journal of Dermatology, 143(6)*, 1248-60.	C
McKenzie, F., White, C.A., Kendall, S., Finlayson, A., Urquhart, M. & Williams, I. (2006). Psychological impact of colostomy pouch change and disposal. *British Journal of Nursing, 15(6)*, 308-316.	D
Millan, M. (2009). Preoperative stoma siting and education by stomatherapists of colorectal cancer patients: a descriptive study in twelve Spanish colorectal units. *Colorectal Disease, 12(7)*, 88-92. doi:10.1111/j.1463-1318.2009.01942.X.	B
Nazarko, L. (2008). Caring for a patient with a urostomy in a community setting. *British Journal of Community Nursing, 13(8)*, 354-361.	D
Nederlandse Stomavereniging (2008). *De kwaliteit van de stomazorg in patiëntenperspectief. Een set van kwaliteitscriteria.* Maarssen: Nederlandse Stomavereniging. Bekkers, M.	D
Nederlandse Stomavereniging (2009a). *Stomagerelateerde complicaties. Onderzoeksverslag in opdracht van de NSV.* Amsterdam: Newcom Research & Consultancy B.V. Kapteijns, A. & Buitinga, S.	C
Nederlandse Stomavereniging (2009b). *De invloed van de stoma op het dagelijks leven. Onderzoeksverslag in opdracht van de NSV.* Amsterdam: Newcom Research & Consultancy B.V. Kapteijns, A. & Buitinga, S.	C
Nederlandse Stomavereniging (2009c). *Kwaliteit en organisatie van stomazorg. Onderzoeksverslag in opdracht van de NSV.* Amsterdam: Newcom Research & Consultancy B.V. Kapteijns, A. & Buitinga, S.	C
Nederlandse Stomavereniging (2010a). *In gesprek over de kwaliteit van de stomazorg.* Maarssen: Nederlandse Stomavereniging Eikelboom, N.I.	D
Nederlandse Stomavereniging (2010b). *Onderzoek naar het gebruik van stomamaterialen. Onderzoeksverslag in opdracht van de NSV.* Amsterdam: Newcom Research & Consultancy B.V. Kapteijns, A., Buitinga, S. & Meeusen, K.	C
Nederlandse Vereniging voor Heelkunde (2011). Normen voor chirurgische behandeling. Verkregen op 31-3-2012 <<*www.kwaliteitskoepel.nl/assets/structured-files/Normen/*>>	D
Needleman, J., Buerhaus, P., Mattke, S., Stewart, M. & Zelevinsky, k., (2002). Nurse staffing levels and the quality of care in hospitals. *The New England Journal of Medicine. 346(22,)* 1715-22. Verkregen op 10-8-2012 nejm.org	B
Nordström, G.M. & Nyman, C.R. (1991). Living with a urostomy. A follow up with special regard to the peristomal-skin complications, psychosocial and sexual life.	C

Scandinavian Journal of Urol. Nephrol. Suppl., 138, 247-251.	
Northouse, L.L., Schafer, J.A., Tipton, J. & Metivier, L. (1999). The concerns of patients and spouses after the diagnosis of colon cancer: a qualitative analysis. *Journal of Wound Ostomy Continence Nursing, 26(1)*, 8-17.	+
Nybaek, H., Bang Knudsen, D., Norgaard Laursen, T., Karlsmark, T. J. & Jemec, G.B.E. (2009). Skin problems in ostomy patients: a case-control study of risk factors. *Acta Derm Venereol, 89(1)*, 64-67. doi: 10.2340/00015555-0536.	C
O'Connor, G. (2005). Teaching stoma-management skills: the importance of selfcare. *British Journal of Nursing, 14(4)*, 320-324.	D
O'Shea, H.S. (2001). Teaching the adult ostomy patient. *Journal of Wound Ostomy Continence Nursing, 28(1)*, 47-54.	D
Park, J.J., Del Pino, A., Orsay, C.P., Nelson, R.L., Pearl, L.K., Cintron, J.R. & Abcarian, H. (1999). Stoma complications: the Cook County Hospital experience. *Diseases of the Colon & Rectum, 42(12)*, 1575-1580.	C
Persson, E., Gustavsson, B., Hellström, A.L., Fridstedt, G., Lappas, G. & Hultén, L. (2005a). Information to the relatives of people with ostomies. *Journal of Wound Ostomy Continence Nursing, 32(4)*, 238-245.	C
Persson, E., Gustavsson, B., Hellström, A.L., Lappas, G. & Hultén, L. (2005b). Ostomy patients' perceptions of quality of care. *Journal of Advanced Nursing, 49(1)*, 51-58.	C
Pieper, B. & Mikols, C. (1996). Predischarge and postdischarge concerns of persons with an ostomy. *Journal of Wound Ostomy Continence Nursing, 23(2)*, 105-109.	C
Pilgrim, C.H.C., McIntyre, R. & Bailey, M. (2010). Prospective audit of parastomal hernia: prevalence and associated comorbidities. *Diseases of the Colon & Rectum, 53(1)*, 71-76. doi: 10.1007/DCR.0b013e3181bdee8c.	B
PON (2006). *Parastomale hernia en hulpmiddelengebruik.* Tilburg: PON Rietveld, T. & Erp, S. van	D
Pontieri-Lewis, V. (2006). Basics of ostomy care. *Med. Surg. Nursing, 15(4)*, 199-202.	D
Poritz, L.S., Lebo, M.A., Bobb, A.D., Ardell, C.M. & Koltun,W.A. (2008). Management of peristomal pyoderma gangrenosum. *Journal of the American College of Surgeons, 206*, 311-315. doi:10.1016/j.jamcollsurg.2007.07.023.	C
Potter, K.L. (2000). Surgical oncology of the pelvis: ostomy planning and management. *Journal of Surgical Oncology, 73(4)*, 237-242.	D
Pringle, W. & Swan, E. (2001). Continuing care after discharge from hospital for stoma patients. *British Journal of Nursing, 10(19)*, 1275-1288.	C
Ratliff, C.R. & Donovan, A.M. (2001). Frequency of peristomal complications. *Ostomy wound management, 47(8)*, 26-29.	C
Ratliff, C.R., Scarano, K.A. & Donovan, A.M. (2005). Descriptive study of peristomal complications. *Journal of Wound Ostomy Continence Nursing, 32(1)*, 33-37.	C
Readding, L.A. (2005). Hospital to home, smoothing the journey for the new ostomist. *British Journal of Nursing, 14(16)*, 16-20.	D
Redmond, C., Cowin, C. & Parker, T. (2009). The experience of faecal leakage among ileostomists. *British Journal of Nursing, 18(17)*, 12-17.	C
Registered nurses' association of Ontario. (2009). *Ostomy care and management. Clinical best practice guidelines.* Ontario: RNAO. Verkregen op 14-2-2011	AGREE

www.rnao.org/bestpractices	
Reynaud, S.N. & Meeker, B.J. (2002). Coping styles of older adults with ostomies. *Journal of Gerontological Nursing, 28(5),* 30 -36.	C
Richbourg, L., Thorpe, J.M. & Rapp, C.G. (2007). Difficulties experienced by the ostomate after hospital discharge. *Journal of Wound Ostomy Continence Nursing, 34(1),* 70-79.	C
Rolstad, B.S. & Erwin-Toth, P.L. (2010). Peristomal skin complications: prevention and management. *American Journal of Nursing, 110(2),* 43-48.	D
Ross, L., Abild-Nielsen, A.G., Thomsen, B.L., Karlsen, R.V., Boesen, E.H. & Johansen, C. (2006). Quality of life of Danish colorectal cancer patients with and without a stoma. *Support Care Cancer, 15(5),* 505-513. doi:10.1007/s00520-006-0177-8	B
Rozen, B.L. (1997). The value of a well-placed stoma. *Cancer Practice, 5(6),* 347-352.	D
Rudoni, C. & Dennis, H. (2009). Accessories or necessities? Exploring consensus on usage of stoma accessories. *British Journal of Nursing, 18(18),* 1106-1112.	++
Salvadalena, G. (2008). Incidence of complications of the stoma and peristomal skin among individuals with colostomy, ileostomy, and urostomy: a systematic review. *Journal of Wound Ostomy Continence Nursing, 35(6),* 596-607.	C
Sica, J. & Burch, J. (2007). Management of intestinal failure and high-output stomas. *British Journal of Nursing, 16(13),* 772- 777.	D
Simmons, K.L., Smith, J.A., Bobb, KA. & Liles, L.L.M. (2007). Adjustment to colostomy: stoma acceptance, stoma care self-efficacy and interpersonal relationships. *Journal of Advanced Nursing, 60(6),* 627-635.	C
Spier, B.J., Fayyad, A.A., Lucey, M.R., Johnson, E.A., Wojtowycz, M., Rikkers, H., Harms, B.A. & Reichelderfer, M. (2008). Bleeding stomal varices: case series and systematic review of the literature. *Clinical Gastroenterology and Hepatology, 6,* 346-352. doi: 10.1016/j.cgh.2007.12.047.	C
Sredl, D. & Aukamp, V. (2006). Evidence-based nursing care management for the pregnant women with an ostomy. *Journal of Wound Ostomy Continence Nursing, 33(1),* 42-49.	D
Thorpe, G., McArthur, M. & Richardson, B. (2009). Bodily change following faecal stoma formation: qualitative interpretive synthesis. *Journal of Advanced Nursing, Review Paper, 65(9),* 1778-1789. doi:10.1111/j.1365-2648.2009.05059.X.	++
Tseng, HC., Wang, HH., Hsu, YY. & Weng, WC. (2004). Factors related to stress in outpatients with permanent colostomies. *Kaohsiung J. Med. Sci., 20(2),* 70-77.	C
Tsukada, K., Tokunaga, K., Iwama, T., Mishima, Y., Tazawa, K. & Fujimaki, M. (1994) Cranberry juice and its impact on peri-stomal skin conditions for urostomy patients. *Ostomy Wound Management, 40(9),* 60-68.	C
Turnbull, G.B. (2002). The ostomy files: the position on preoperative stoma site positioning. *Vancouver Ostomy High Life, 41(1),* 1,14.	D
Turnbull, G.B. (2003). A look at the purpose and outcomes of colostomy irrigation. *Ostomy Wound Management, 49(2),*19-20.	D
Vink, M. (2007). De obese patiënte en stomazorg. *WCS Nieuws, 24(1),* 45-47.	D
Vujnovich, A. (2008). Pre and post- operative assessment of patients with a stoma. *Nursing Standard, 22(19),* 50-56.	D

Welink- Lamberts B., Werkgroep CHIODAZ (2007). Nieuwe dieetbehandelingsrichtlijn ileostoma. *Ned. Tijdschrift voor Voeding & Diëtiek 62(3),* 7-10.	D
Williams, J. (2007). Stoma care nursing: what the community nurse needs to know. *British Journal of Community Nursing, 12(8),* 342- 346.	D
Woo, K.Y., Sibbald, R.G., Ayello, E.A., Coutts, P.M. & Garde, D.E. (2009). Peristomal Skin Complications and Management. *Advanced in Skin & Wound Care, 22(11),* 522-532.	D
Wound Ostomy and Continence Nurses Society (2010). *Management of the patient with a fecal ostomy: Best practice guideline for clinicals.* Mount Laurel: Wound Ostomy and Continence Nurses Society (NJ) Goldberg, M., Aukett, L.K., Carmel, J., Fellows, J. & Pittman, J.	AGREE
Wu, H.K.M., Chau, J.PC. & Twinn, S., (2007). Self-efficacy and quality of life among stoma patients in Hong Kong. *Cancer Nursing, 30(3),* 186-193.	C
Yeo,H., Abir, F., Longo, W.E. (2006). Management of parastomal ulcers. *World Journal of Gastroenterology, 12(20),* 3133-3137.	D